SUCCESSFUL INTERMITTENT FASTING FOR WOMEN OVER 50

SIMPLE STEPS TO HELP YOU LOSE WEIGHT, BOOST METABOLISM, CLEAR BRAIN FOG, AND INCREASE ENERGY TO LIVE A HEALTHIER LIFE WITHOUT FEELING HUNGRY

JENNIFER LINDSEY

Copyright © 2024 Jennifer Lindsey. All rights reserved.

The content within this book may not be reproduced, duplicated, or transmitted without direct written permission from the author or the publisher.

Under no circumstances will any blame or legal responsibility be held against the publisher, or author, for any damages, reparation, or monetary loss due to the information contained within this book, either directly or indirectly.

Legal Notice:

This book is copyright protected. It is only for personal use. You cannot amend, distribute, sell, use, quote, or paraphrase any part of the content within this book, without the consent of the author or publisher.

Disclaimer Notice:

Please note the information contained within this document is for educational and entertainment purposes only. All effort has been expended to present accurate, up-to-date, reliable, and complete information. No warranties of any kind are declared or implied. Readers acknowledge that the author is not engaged in the rendering of legal, financial, medical, or professional advice. The content within this book has been derived from various sources. Please consult a licensed professional before attempting any techniques outlined in this book.

By reading this document, the reader agrees that under no circumstances is the author responsible for any losses, direct or indirect, that are incurred as a result of the use of the information contained within this document, including, but not limited to, errors, omissions, or inaccuracies.

CONTENTS

Introduction   7

1. UNDERSTANDING INTERMITTENT FASTING AND ITS BENEFITS   11
   1.1 What is Intermittent Fasting? A Comprehensive Overview   11
   1.2 Decoding the Science: How Intermittent Fasting Affects Metabolism After 50   13
   1.3 Autophagy and Aging: Why IF is Especially Beneficial Post-Menopause   15
   1.4 Addressing Common Myths and Misconceptions About Intermittent Fasting   18
   1.5 Hormonal Changes and IF: Tailoring Your Fasting Strategy   20
   1.6 The Impact of Intermittent Fasting on Mental Clarity and Focus   23

2. PREPARING FOR INTERMITTENT FASTING   27
   2.1 Assessing Your Health: When to Consult a Professional   27
   2.2 Transitioning Smoothly: Gradual Steps to Start Intermittent Fasting   29
   2.3 Managing Expectations: Realistic Goals and Timelines   31
   2.4 Nutritional Guidelines to Follow Before Starting IF   33
   2.5 The Importance of Hydration During Fasting Periods   35
   2.6 Mental Preparation: Building a Resilient Mindset   37

3. INTERMITTENT FASTING METHODS AND SCHEDULES   41
   3.1 Exploring Different Fasting Windows: 16/8, 5:2, and More   41
   3.2 Time-Restricted Eating: A Day in the Life   45
   3.3 The 5:2 Method: Detailed Weekly Plan   47

3.4 The Eat Stop Eat Method: Detailed Weekly Plan	49
3.5 Pros and Cons of Spontaneous Meal Skipping	52
3.6 Customizing Your Fasting Plan: Adjustments for Energy and Hunger	54
3.7 Combining Intermittent Fasting with Other Diets	57
4. NUTRITION AND MEAL PLANNING	61
4.1 Essential Nutrients and Supplements for Women Over 50	61
4.2 Building a Menopause-Friendly Meal Plan	64
4.3 Easy and Nutritional Recipes for Non-Fasting Days	66
4.4 Smart Snacking: What to Eat During Your Eating Window	69
4.5 Preparing Meals for One: Tips and Tricks	71
4.6 Integrating Family Meals with Your IF Schedule	74
5. INTERMITTENT FASTING FRIENDLY RECIPES	79
5.1 Healthy Snack Options	80
5.2 Breakfasts	84
5.3 Lunch	88
5.4 Dinner	91
5.5 Meals that are Only 500 to 800 Calories	94
5.6 Daily Meal Plan: 500 to 600 Calories	99
5.7 Daily Meal Plan: 600 to 800 Calories	101
5.8 Daily Meal Plan: 800 to 1000 Calories	103
6. OVERCOMING CHALLENGES AND SETBACKS	107
6.1 Handling Hunger Pangs: Tips and Tricks	107
6.2 Social Eating and Intermittent Fasting: How to Balance Both	110
6.3 Dealing with Plateaus: Next Steps When Weight Loss Stalls	112
6.4 Adjusting Your Fasting Schedule Around Medical Needs	115
6.5 Emotional Eating vs. Scheduled Eating: Establishing Control	117
6.6 Fasting During Holidays and Special Occasions	119

7. **PHYSICAL ACTIVITY AND INTERMITTENT FASTING** — 123
   - 7.1 The Best Types of Exercise to Pair with Intermittent Fasting — 123
   - 7.2 Low-Impact Workouts for Sustainable Health — 126
   - 7.3 Yoga and Mindfulness: Enhancing Mental and Physical Health — 128
   - 7.4 Scheduling Workouts: Best Times During Your Fasting Cycle — 131
   - 7.5 Avoiding Overexertion: Listening to Your Body's Signals — 134
   - 7.6 Incorporating Regular Movement into Your Routine — 136

8. **LONG-TERM STRATEGIES FOR SUCCESS** — 139
   - 8.1 Developing a Long-Term Mindset: Beyond Quick Fixes — 139
   - 8.2 Adapting IF Practices as You Age — 141
   - 8.3 Keeping a Journal: Tracking Your Progress and Reflections — 143
   - 8.4 Community and Support: Finding Like-Minded Individuals — 146
   - 8.5 Continuous Learning: Keeping Up-to-Date with IF Research — 148
   - 8.6 When to Reevaluate Your IF Approach — 150

9. **SUCCESS STORIES AND INSPIRATIONAL INSIGHTS** — 153
   - 9.1 Transformative Tales: Women Over 50 Who Thrived with IF — 153
   - 9.2 Expert Opinions: Why Doctors Recommend IF for Aging Women — 156
   - 9.3 Overcoming Health Hurdles with Intermittent Fasting — 158
   - 9.4 Mental Health Improvements from Real IF Practitioners — 160
   - 9.5 The Role of IF in Longevity and Disease Prevention — 162
   - 9.6 Celebrating Your Success: Embracing a Healthier, Happier You — 165

Conclusion 169
Glossary 173
References 177

INTRODUCTION

Three years ago, Helen, a vibrant woman in her early fifties, found herself at a crossroads. Despite her best efforts, the scale refused to budge, her mind seemed shrouded in fog, and her energy levels had dipped lower than she ever thought possible. During this frustrating season of life, she stumbled upon intermittent fasting. Skeptical yet desperate for a change, Helen decided to give it a try. To her amazement, not only did she start losing weight, but her mental clarity improved, and her vitality began to soar. Helen's story is not unique; it mirrors the experiences of countless women over 50 who have discovered the rejuvenating power of this simple yet effective lifestyle tweak.

Intermittent fasting is more than just a diet trend; it's a sustainable approach to eating that has been embraced by millions seeking a healthier lifestyle. Unlike rigid dieting routines that are hard to maintain, intermittent fasting offers flexibility and adaptability, making it particularly appealing to those of us over 50 who face unique dietary challenges.

As we age, our bodies experience profound transformations. The ebb and flow of hormones, coupled with a gradual deceleration in our metabolism, often render conventional diets less effective and, frankly, disheartening. It's crucial to recognize that our nutritional needs and how our bodies metabolize food evolve over time. Enter intermittent fasting: a revolutionary approach that rejuvenates our body's metabolic processes and fine-tunes hormone regulation.

This book is crafted with you in mind, aiming to demystify intermittent fasting and tailor it to meet the specific needs and challenges faced by women over 50. From uncovering the science behind fasting to offering personalized fasting strategies, this guide covers it all. You'll find practical advice on how to integrate this approach into your life, alongside motivational insights to keep you inspired.

The benefits of intermittent fasting extend well beyond weight loss. Many women report enhanced mental clarity, increased energy levels, and an overall boost in well-being. Scientific studies and authentic experiences shared by women like you support these advantages. Moving forward, we will explore these benefits in greater detail, unveiling the scientific evidence and sharing inspiring stories from women who have witnessed the transformative effects of intermittent fasting firsthand.

My journey into writing this book began from a deep-seated desire to help women like Helen, perhaps like you, reclaim their health and vitality in midlife and beyond. Drawing from my extensive experience in nutrition and food, along with valuable lessons learned from personal endeavors, I am uniquely positioned to guide you through this transformative journey. My background, enriched by both professional and personal experiences, has equipped me to navigate you through this transformative process with understanding and care.

In the following chapters, we'll take a step-by-step look at how to adopt intermittent fasting into your life. You'll learn about the different types of fasting plans, how to handle potential challenges, and the best ways to combine fasting with nutritious eating. This book is designed to be both informative and easy to navigate, ensuring you feel supported every step of the way.

As you turn these pages, I encourage you to keep an open mind and consider how these principles could be adapted to fit your lifestyle and health goals. Remember, it's never too late to embrace change and experience a new level of health and vitality.

I invite you to not just read this book but to engage actively with it. Consider keeping a journal of your fasting journey, noting how you feel and the changes you see. Let this book serve as your guide and companion as you discover the empowering world of intermittent fasting for women over 50. Let's begin this journey together, shall we?

UNDERSTANDING INTERMITTENT FASTING AND ITS BENEFITS

Have you ever felt that despite your best efforts, the old ways of managing your weight and health just don't seem to work anymore? You're not alone. Like many women over 50, you might find yourself wrestling with unyielding scales and dwindling energy levels. But what if there was a way to reignite your metabolism, clear the mental fog, and boost your energy without resorting to restrictive diets that feel more punishing than beneficial? This is where intermittent fasting steps in—a lifestyle strategy that has brought new hope and real results to many.

1.1 WHAT IS INTERMITTENT FASTING? A COMPREHENSIVE OVERVIEW

Intermittent fasting (IF) isn't about which foods to eat but focuses on when you eat. It involves cycling between periods of eating and fasting. It's not a diet in the traditional sense but rather a pattern of eating that has helped many regain control over their health. The most popular methods include:

- The 16/8 method, where you fast for 16 hours and eat during an 8-hour window.
- The 5:2 method involves eating normally five days a week while restricting calories for two non-consecutive days.
- Eat-Stop-Eat, which entails fasting for 24 hours once or twice a week.

Other methods of IF include:

- Alternate day fasting, which involves fasting every other day.
- Warrior Diet: Eat small amounts of raw fruits and vegetables during the day and one large meal at night.
- 24-Hour Fast, fasting for 24 hours once or twice a week.
- Spontaneous Meal Skipping: skipping meals occasionally based on convenience or lack of hunger.
- OMAD (One Meal A Day) involves fasting for 23 hours and consuming all calories in one large meal within one hour.

Historically, fasting isn't new. It has been practiced in various forms for millennia, often for religious or spiritual reasons. Today's intermittent fasting draws on these age-old traditions, modernized for contemporary health goals. Its roots in ancient practices help explain why it feels more sustainable—more in tune with our bodies' natural rhythms than the latest diet fads.

The simplicity and flexibility of intermittent fasting have contributed to its rising popularity, particularly among women in their fifties and beyond. This age group appreciates that intermittent fasting doesn't require overhauling what is eaten but rather when food is consumed, making it a manageable and

UNDERSTANDING INTERMITTENT FASTING AND ITS BENEFI... | 13

adaptable approach amidst the busy, often unpredictable life schedules typical of this stage.

Contrasting sharply with traditional diets that focus heavily on calorie restriction and meticulous control over food intake, intermittent fasting offers a liberating approach to weight loss and health enhancement. Instead of counting every calorie, it empowers you to focus on timing, which naturally leads to reduced calorie intake without the need to micromanage every meal. This shift not only helps in managing weight but also aligns well with your body's needs, accommodating the natural changes in metabolism that occur with age.

Interactive Element: Reflective Journal Prompt

To help integrate the concept of intermittent fasting into your life, consider keeping a reflective journal. Start by answering this question in your journal: "What are my initial thoughts and feelings about adopting an intermittent fasting approach? What method might suit my lifestyle and why?" Reflecting on these questions can help clarify your thoughts and set a purposeful intention as you explore intermittent fasting further.

1.2 DECODING THE SCIENCE: HOW INTERMITTENT FASTING AFFECTS METABOLISM AFTER 50

Transitioning into our fifties and beyond, we often notice that our bodies react differently than they did in our younger years. Notably, our metabolic rates—the mechanisms by which our bodies convert food and beverages into usable energy—start to slow. This deceleration is prominently observed post-menopause, as estrogen levels take a sharp dive, affecting the way our bodies process carbohydrates and sugars. Additionally, aging is commonly accompanied by reduced muscle mass, further slowing our metabolism since muscles are more efficient at burning calories than fat. These natural changes can complicate weight management efforts, leading to potential weight gain despite maintaining previous dietary habits. Here, intermittent fasting emerges as a transformative strategy, leveraging these age-related metabolic shifts to our advantage.

Intermittent fasting can influence your metabolism in several beneficial ways. One of the most significant effects is its ability to improve insulin sensitivity. Insulin is a hormone that allows your cells to absorb glucose, a type of sugar that serves as a critical energy source. As sensitivity improves, your body becomes better at processing glucose, which can help manage blood sugar levels more efficiently. This is crucial as we age, given the increased risk for type 2 diabetes and other metabolic health issues. Intermittent fasting boosts norepinephrine production, a hormone instrumental in the fat-burning process. This enhancement is especially advantageous for individuals facing a deceleration in metabolism due to aging.

Several studies underscore the benefits of intermittent fasting on metabolism, particularly in older adults. For instance, research published in the journal' Cell Metabolism' showed that intermittent fasting could increase metabolic rate and aid in weight loss by enhancing hormone function and boosting fat-burning processes, even in post-menopausal women. These studies are pivotal as they translate the theoretical benefits of intermittent fasting into tangible outcomes, demonstrating that age does not diminish the potential metabolic advantages of this eating pattern.

When it comes to adapting intermittent fasting to fit individual metabolic needs, it's crucial to start slowly and listen to your body. Each person's metabolic response to fasting will differ. Some may find that shorter fasting periods, for example, the 16/8 method, which involves fasting for sixteen hours and eating during an eight-hour window, often proves to be a balanced approach that yields considerable benefits without placing undue stress on the body. Others might explore the 5:2 approach, reducing calorie intake two days a week, which can also positively impact metabolic health without the rigidity of daily fasting. It's about finding a rhythm that feels sustainable and responsive to your body's signals, like adjusting your eating window to earlier in the day to align with natural circadian rhythms, which can further enhance metabolic efficiency.

Navigating these changes requires patience and experimentation. It's also wise to keep a record of how you feel during different fasting schedules to fine-tune what works best for your lifestyle and health goals. This personalized approach ensures that intermittent fasting remains a viable and effective strategy for managing metabolism and overall health as we age.

1.3 AUTOPHAGY AND AGING: WHY IF IS ESPECIALLY BENEFICIAL POST-MENOPAUSE

Understanding autophagy and its implications for aging is like uncovering a hidden gem in the quest for maintaining youthfulness and health. Autophagy, a term derived from the Greek words for "self" and "eating," refers to the body's process of cleaning out damaged cells and regenerating newer, healthier ones. This natural recycling mechanism is crucial for cellular health and longevity. It helps clear out protein aggregates, damaged organelles, and pathogens, thereby reducing the likelihood of various age-related diseases.

When we explore the relationship between intermittent fasting and autophagy, it becomes clear why this eating pattern is particularly resonant for those of us navigating the post-menopausal phase of life. Intermittent fasting has been shown to trigger significant increases in autophagy. Fasting provides a kind of stress that prompts our cells to enhance their internal cleaning processes. It's akin to giving the body a much-needed rest from the constant work of digestion and nutrient assimilation, allowing it to focus instead on maintenance and repair. This is particularly beneficial as our cells age and naturally accumulate more damage. By enhancing autophagy, intermittent fasting helps to mitigate the effects of cellular aging, contributing to better health and disease prevention.

The benefits of this process are particularly profound for post-menopausal women. As estrogen levels decline with menopause, the risk of various age-related diseases increases. Enhanced autophagy can help counteract these risks by improving cellular function and resilience. For instance, better autophagy is linked to reduced inflammation, a key factor in many chronic diseases, including heart disease and diabetes, which tend to appear more frequently in later life. Additionally, by removing damaged cellular components, autophagy plays a role in preventing cancer, which becomes an increasing concern with age. The cellular housekeeping facilitated by autophagy not only helps slow the aging process but also enhances the body's ability to repair itself, thereby improving overall vitality and extending health span.

The research underscores the role of intermittent fasting in boosting autophagy among older women, providing a solid scientific foundation for its benefits. A study published in the

'Aging Research Reviews highlighted that intermittent fasting could induce autophagy across various organs, which is critical for metabolism regulation and cellular stress resilience. This is particularly important for aging women who experience a natural decline in cellular function. Another significant research finding from the 'Journal of Molecular and Cellular Endocrinology' reported that intermittent fasting could adjust cellular mechanisms like autophagy, which helps in adapting to post-menopausal changes in the body, thereby aiding in weight management and metabolic health.

These studies are pivotal, not just for their scientific merit but for the practical hope they offer. They suggest that by incorporating intermittent fasting into our lives, we can proactively enhance our body's ability to maintain cellular health through autophagy. This isn't just about increasing lifespan, but about enriching our later years with better health and vitality. It's about giving our bodies the tools they need to naturally fight the wear and tear of aging, allowing us to lead fuller, more active lives even as we age.

For those of us looking to integrate intermittent fasting into our lives to enhance autophagy, it's important to approach this transition with mindfulness and patience. Starting with shorter fasting periods and gradually increasing the duration as the body adapts can make the process more manageable. It's also crucial to pay attention to the body's signals and to consult healthcare providers to tailor the fasting routine to personal health needs and conditions. This personalized approach ensures not only the effectiveness of the fasting routine but also its sustainability in the long term, paving the way for a healthier approach to aging.

1.4 ADDRESSING COMMON MYTHS AND MISCONCEPTIONS ABOUT INTERMITTENT FASTING

As we explore the realm of intermittent fasting, it's crucial to clear the fog surrounding some of the most common myths. Often, misinformation can lead to unnecessary concerns that might deter someone from trying this potentially life-altering approach. Let's set the record straight and ensure you have the facts to make an informed decision about whether intermittent fasting is right for you.

One of the most pervasive myths is that intermittent fasting leads to muscle loss. This concern is understandable; after all, it seems logical that not eating for extended periods might cause your body to consume muscle for energy. However, research tells a different story. Intermittent fasting can actually be muscle-sparing if done correctly. When you fast, human growth hormone levels increase, and insulin levels decrease. This environment allows your body to preferentially burn fat for energy rather than muscle. Muscle degradation typically happens when the body has no access to fat and must turn to muscle for energy, a scenario unlikely to occur in well-planned intermittent fasting. For added muscle protection, incorporating a routine of resistance training can be highly beneficial, promoting muscle growth and maintenance even as you fast.

Another common concern is the difference between hunger and starvation, a distinction that is vital to understand. Hunger during intermittent fasting is normal and can be seen as a sign that your body is adjusting to new eating schedules. It's typically mild and temporary, often disappearing as your body adapts to the fasting routine. On the other hand, starvation is a severe deficiency in caloric intake and essential nutrients over an extended period. Intermittent fasting, when followed correctly, does not lead to starvation; you still consume all the necessary nutrients within your eating windows, just at different times of the day. This adjustment period is crucial, and keeping hydrated and busy during fasting hours can help mitigate feelings of hunger.

Misconceptions about the health benefits of intermittent fasting also need addressing. While IF offers numerous health benefits, it's not a cure-all. It's important to approach fasting with realistic expectations. Intermittent fasting has been shown to aid in weight loss, improve metabolic health, and reduce inflammation. Still, it may not have the same effects for everyone and is not suitable for certain health conditions without professional guidance. It's vital to consult healthcare providers to tailor the fasting approach to individual health needs, particularly if you have pre-existing conditions such as diabetes or heart issues.

Lastly, let's tackle the worries about feeling weak or unable to concentrate during fasting periods. These concerns are common and can be part of the body's initial response to a new fasting schedule. However, these symptoms often diminish as your body becomes accustomed to the new routine. To ease these effects, it's helpful to start with shorter fasting periods and gradually increase as you feel more comfortable. Ensuring you stay hydrated and consume nutrient-rich foods during your eating windows can also play a significant role in maintaining energy levels and mental clarity.

It is also important to remember to stay hydrated during your fasting periods, you can drink during intermittent fasting windows, but it's important to choose beverages that do not break your fast. Here are the types of drinks that are typically allowed during fasting periods:

- Water: Essential for hydration and can be consumed freely. Plain or sparkling water is fine.
- Black Coffee: Contains very few calories and can help suppress appetite. Avoid adding sugar, cream, or milk.
- Tea: Similar to coffee, plain tea (black, green, or herbal) is acceptable as long as it doesn't contain added sugars or calories.
- Apple Cider Vinegar or Lemon: Some people add a small amount of apple cider vinegar or lemon to water for potential health benefits.

It's important to avoid any beverages that contain calories, sugars, or artificial sweeteners, as these can break your fast and impact the benefits of intermittent fasting.

Remember, intermittent fasting is flexible; finding a pattern that fits your lifestyle and listening to your body's responses is critical to sustaining this practice without feeling deprived or overly stressed.

By debunking these myths and understanding the realities of intermittent fasting, you can approach this dietary strategy with confidence and clarity. Remember, knowledge is power, and being well-informed will help you navigate the initial challenges and reap the significant health benefits intermittent fasting can offer.

1.5 HORMONAL CHANGES AND IF: TAILORING YOUR FASTING STRATEGY

Navigating through your fifties introduces a cascade of hormonal changes that significantly impact your health and weight. The decline of estrogen and progesterone levels during and after menopause can lead to a slower metabolism, weight gain, especially around the abdomen, and increased risk of heart disease and osteoporosis. These hormonal shifts can also influence insulin sensitivity, which affects how your body processes sugar and can lead to higher blood sugar levels. It's a pivotal time to reconsider how you support your body, and intermittent fasting (IF) can be a powerful tool in managing these hormonal upheavals.

Intermittent fasting's impact on hormonal health is profound, particularly its ability to stabilize insulin levels and improve overall hormone sensitivity. When you fast, your insulin levels decrease, which not only helps prevent spikes in blood sugar but also reduces insulin resistance, a common issue as we age. This adjustment can lead to improved metabolic health and reduced risk of type 2 diabetes, a concern that grows with hormonal changes post-menopause. Moreover, fasting increases human growth hormone levels, which helps in fat-burning and muscle growth, countering the muscle loss often associated with aging. This hormonal regulation is critical for maintaining a balanced and healthy body as you navigate through your fifties and beyond.

Tailoring intermittent fasting to fit hormonal needs requires a thoughtful approach. For many women, the length of the fasting window can be critical. You might find that shorter fasting periods, such as 14-16 hours, are more manageable and still yield significant benefits. For others, tweaking the timing of the eating window to earlier in the day to align with natural circadian rhythms can enhance hormone balance and improve sleep quality, which in itself can help regulate other hormones like cortisol, known for its role in stress and metabolism.

Let's consider the experiences of real women who have adapted intermittent fasting to their lives amidst hormonal changes. Maria, a 53-year-old teacher, started practicing the 16/8 method after entering menopause. She noticed a reduction in her midsection weight and significant improvements in her energy levels and sleep patterns. Maria's case illustrates the importance of adjusting fasting times; she preferred having her eating window close by 6 PM, which significantly improved her sleep, a common issue during menopause due to hormonal fluctuations.

Another compelling case is Susan, a 57-year-old retired banker who opted for the 5:2 method. She manages her calorie intake two days a week, which has helped her handle her prediabetic state more effectively. Susan appreciated that this method reduced the rigidity of daily fasting, which she found too daunting. Her approach demonstrates the flexibility of IF in managing health through dietary adjustments without the need for daily restrictions.

These anecdotes underscore the potential of intermittent fasting to adapt to the unique hormonal needs of women over 50. By understanding your body's signals and being open to adjustments, you can find a fasting rhythm that addresses weight management and enhances your overall hormonal health. Whether it's choosing which type of intermittent fasting method to follow or deciding the duration of fasts, the critical is to listen to your body and make informed choices that support your health at this stage of life.

As we continue to explore the relationship between diet, lifestyle, and hormonal health, it becomes clear that intermittent fasting offers more than just a way to manage weight—it provides a pathway to enhance overall well-being and vitality during a time of significant change. The flexibility to adapt your fasting schedule as you learn more about your body's responses makes intermittent fasting a practical approach and a sustainable one, offering benefits that extend beyond the scale.

1.6 THE IMPACT OF INTERMITTENT FASTING ON MENTAL CLARITY AND FOCUS

Imagine waking up on a morning when the fog in your brain lifts faster than the mist over a serene lake. Where your thoughts align with clarity and precision, allowing you to tackle your daily tasks with renewed energy and focus. This isn't just a pleasant daydream for many women over 50 who practice intermittent fasting; it's a delightful reality. The cognitive benefits of intermittent fasting stretch beyond mere weight management, touching on aspects of mental clarity and enhanced focus that are especially beneficial as we age.

The science behind these mental enhancements is as fascinating as the outcomes are beneficial. One of the key players in this process is the Brain-Derived Neurotrophic Factor (BDNF), a protein that acts as fertilizer for your brain, encouraging the growth of new neurons and helping protect existing ones. Intermittent fasting boosts the production of BDNF, effectively giving your brain a mini-renovation. This increase in BDNF not only helps with current cognitive function but also adds a layer of protection against various neurodegenerative diseases.

Further contributing to mental clarity is the reduction in inflammation that often accompanies intermittent fasting. Chronic inflammation is like a smoldering fire in the body that, over time, can damage healthy cells and tissues. By reducing inflammation, intermittent fasting helps to preserve the integrity of brain cells, leading to improved cognitive functions. It's akin to clearing the weeds in your garden so that the flowers can bloom more brightly.

For those looking to maximize these cognitive benefits, the timing of your fasting and eating windows plays a crucial role. Aligning your eating window with your body's natural circadian rhythms can enhance mental clarity further. For example, ending your eating window early in the evening can lead to better sleep quality, which is crucial for cognitive function. Hydration, too, plays a significant role. During fasting periods, maintaining adequate hydration is vital. Dehydration can lead to brain fog and fatigue, counteracting the very benefits you seek from fasting. Including electrolyte-rich beverages like coconut water or adding a pinch of Himalayan salt to your water can help maintain electrolyte balance and support better brain function.

Many women who have integrated intermittent fasting into their lives after 50 share stories of transformation that include not just a physical change but a mental revival. Take Ellen, for example, a 55-year-old school principal who started intermittent fasting as a way to manage her weight. What she didn't anticipate was the profound impact it would have on her work life. Ellen reports that her ability to concentrate during long meetings and make decisive, clear-headed decisions has significantly improved. This change has not only made her feel more competent but also more confident in her professional role.

Similarly, Janet, a 62-year-old retired librarian, took up intermittent fasting to improve her health but was pleasantly surprised by the boost in her cognitive function. She finds joy in the clarity with which she can now engage in her hobbies, such as crossword puzzles and writing poetry, which were becoming frustrating due to a previously foggy mind. Janet's experience underscores the profound impact that nurturing our brain health can have on our overall quality of life, bringing into focus the activities that bring us joy and fulfilment.

These testimonies highlight a crucial aspect of intermittent fasting that goes beyond physical health metrics. They paint a picture of a lifestyle adjustment that offers a holistic approach to aging — one that considers the health of both body and mind. As we continue to understand and embrace these benefits, intermittent fasting stands out not just as a tool for weight management, but as a key to unlocking a more vibrant, focused, and fulfilling later life.

Staying informed and conscious of how our bodies and minds are interconnected allows us to make lifestyle choices that support overall well-being. With intermittent fasting, the potential to enhance cognitive function is an exciting prospect, giving us not just hope but also the means to maintain mental sharpness and vitality well into our later years. So, as we sip our morning tea and plan our day during our eating window, we can do so knowing that we are nurturing our minds with every thoughtful sip and every planned pause.

PREPARING FOR INTERMITTENT FASTING

Embarking on an intermittent fasting journey can feel like exploring uncharted waters. Just as a captain must be well-versed in navigating the complexities of the ocean, including its conditions, currents, and climatic changes, so too must you be equipped with a comprehensive understanding of your body's specific needs and potential reactions to fasting. It is crucial to approach intermittent fasting with a well-thought-out strategy and a mindset geared towards enhancing your well-being, ensuring that it augments your health rather than detracts from it.

2.1 ASSESSING YOUR HEALTH: WHEN TO CONSULT A PROFESSIONAL

Before diving into the fasting schedule, conducting a thorough health assessment is imperative. This is especially crucial for women over 50, as this demographic may have specific health considerations such as hormonal changes due to menopause, pre-existing conditions, or medications that could influence how you approach fasting. Understanding your current health status is akin to a pilot performing a pre-flight check—it's essential for ensuring a safe and compelling journey.

Begin by evaluating your overall health, focusing on any chronic conditions you may have, such as diabetes, hypertension, or cardiovascular diseases. These conditions do not automatically disqualify you from practicing intermittent fasting, but they influence the type of fasting schedule that's best for you and may require modifications to your approach. For instance, fasting can significantly affect blood sugar levels, which is particularly relevant for managing diabetes.

Next, consider your current medications. Some require food intake to ensure proper absorption, and others need to be explicitly timed around meals to prevent side effects or interactions. Your medication may need to be adjusted to fit your fasting window, which should be done under the guidance of a healthcare provider.

Consulting with healthcare professionals is an essential step in your preparation. Make appointments to discuss your plan with a general practitioner who understands your medical history, and consider consulting a dietitian or an endocrinologist. These professionals can provide personalized advice based on your health status and help you understand how to integrate fasting into your lifestyle safely. They can also help you identify any potential risks specific to your health conditions and suggest appropriate modifications.

Understanding the contraindications for fasting is crucial. Certain conditions, such as advanced diabetes or severe cardiovascular diseases, may complicate your ability to practice intermittent fasting safely. Your healthcare provider can help you understand these risks and decide whether intermittent fasting is a viable option for you. If it is, they can guide you on approaching it safely.

Finally, regular monitoring and readiness to adjust your fasting plan based on professional feedback are essential. Just as conditions at sea can change, necessitating a course correction, so too can your health needs evolve as you progress with intermittent fasting. Regular check-ups will help you navigate these changes safely and effectively. Keeping a detailed log of your fasting times, dietary intake, and how you feel can be invaluable during these check-ups and provide your healthcare provider with the information needed to tailor advice and adjustments to your plan.

Interactive Element: Journaling Prompt

Maintain a health journal to keep track of your health assessments and any changes in your condition or medication. Start by listing any current health issues, medications, and significant concerns you have about fasting. Note down the advice provided by your healthcare professionals during your consultations, and regularly update this journal with any changes or new insights. This practice will help you stay organized and ensure that you are fully aware of how your body responds to intermittent fasting over time.

2.2 TRANSITIONING SMOOTHLY: GRADUAL STEPS TO START INTERMITTENT FASTING

Embarking on intermittent fasting is much like adapting to a new rhythm in your daily life. It's not just about marking the hours you eat or don't eat; it's about easing your body into a new pattern that feels natural and sustainable. To make this transition as smooth as possible, it's wise to start with less intensive fasting intervals. Think of it as dipping your toes into the water rather than diving headfirst into the deep end. You may begin with a shorter fasting window, fasting for 12 hours and eating over 12 hours. This can be as simple as finishing dinner by 7 PM and then eating breakfast at

7 AM the following day. Such a schedule might not feel drastically different from your current routine but can significantly help your body adjust to periods of not eating.

Gradually, as you feel more comfortable and your body adapts, you can start to extend the fasting period. This doesn't have to happen overnight. In fact, extending the fasting window by just one hour every week or two can make the transition much smoother. For example, if you started with a 12-hour fast, consider moving to 13 hours and gauge how you feel. Listen to your body at each step—how do you feel during the fasting periods? Are you experiencing heightened energy levels or, perhaps, bouts of fatigue? Adjusting the length of your fasting window based on your body's signals is crucial. This gradual increase helps mitigate potential discomforts such as excessive hunger or irritability that can sometimes accompany more abrupt fasting schedules.

The art of listening to your body is perhaps the most crucial skill you can develop during this process. It's about paying attention to both the physical and emotional cues that your body gives you. If you find yourself feeling unusually stressed or fatigued, it might be a sign to ease up and perhaps shorten your fasting window for a while. On the other hand, you might discover an unexpected surge in vitality and clarity—signals that your body is adapting well. **Remember,** intermittent fasting isn't a one-size-fits-all solution; it's a personal tool that you can tailor to fit your unique health needs and lifestyle.

In today's digital age, various tools can help you monitor and adjust your fasting schedule. Mobile apps specifically designed for intermittent fasting can be particularly helpful. These apps often allow you to set fasting and eating windows and will enable you to receive notifications to help keep you on track. Many also offer features that allow you to log your mood and energy levels, providing a comprehensive view of how different fasting intervals affect you. Keeping a journal, either digital or paper, can also be an invaluable aid. Documenting your meals, how you felt during different parts of your fast, and any changes in your physical or emotional well-being can provide insights into the most effective fasting routine for your body. It also serves as a wonderful reflection tool, showing you just how far you've come in your intermittent fasting journey.

By approaching intermittent fasting with a mindset of gradual change, listening deeply to your body's needs, and utilizing tools to track and support your progress, you can ensure a smooth and enjoyable transition. This thoughtful approach not only makes adopting intermittent fasting more manageable but also enhances the sustainability of this practice, allowing you to integrate it effectively into your lifestyle for long-term benefits.

2.3 MANAGING EXPECTATIONS: REALISTIC GOALS AND TIMELINES

Starting something new, like intermittent fasting, is like planting a garden. You wouldn't plant seeds one day and expect a full bloom the next morning. Similarly, setting realistic goals and understanding the growth timeline is vital to nurturing your health through intermittent fasting. It's about cultivating patience and recognizing the smaller victories along the way.

Firstly, let's talk about setting achievable goals. While weight loss might be the most advertised benefit of intermittent fasting, focusing solely on the scale can sometimes lead to disappointment or misjudged efforts. Instead, consider setting goals that are not just about weight loss but also about improving overall health markers. For example, you might aim to stabilize your blood sugar levels, which is especially beneficial if you're managing conditions like prediabetes. Another goal could be to enhance your cardiovascular health by lowering blood pressure or improving your cholesterol profile. These targets provide clear objectives and help you focus on the comprehensive health benefits of intermittent fasting.

Understanding the timeline for these benefits is just as crucial. It's important to know that the body takes time to adjust to new eating patterns and that benefits can accumulate at different rates. Typically, initial changes, such as feeling more energetic during fasting periods or not feeling overly hungry, might be noticed within the first few weeks. More substantial health improvements, like weight loss or better blood sugar control, may take a couple of months to become evident. This timeline can vary widely depending on individual health status, the specific intermittent fasting routine followed, and lifestyle factors such as sleep and stress management.

Recognizing non-scale victories is a key aspect of maintaining motivation and acknowledging progress, particularly when the scale doesn't show immediate changes. These victories can be as simple as feeling more alert in the mornings, experiencing more stable energy levels throughout the day, or finding that you can go longer between meals without feeling hungry. Perhaps you notice an improvement in your sleep quality or that you no longer feel sluggish in the afternoons. Celebrating these small wins not only boosts your morale but also reinforces the positive impact intermittent fasting has on your body beyond weight loss.

Flexibility is a critical component of successful intermittent fasting, much like how gardeners must sometimes relocate plants to better-suited spots. As you progress, you might find the need to adjust your fasting schedule or dietary choices. For instance, if you initially set a goal to lose a certain amount of weight but find yourself feeling drained or irritable, it might be wise to adjust your approach, perhaps by shortening your fasting window or reassessing your nutritional intake during eating periods. Similarly, if you find that your blood sugar levels aren't improving as expected, it might be necessary to consult with a dietitian to further refine your eating plan during non-fasting periods.

Navigating intermittent fasting is a dynamic process, much like navigating life's other challenges. By setting realistic goals, understanding the natural progression of dietary adaptations, celebrating non-scale victories, and being flexible in your approach, you create a sustainable practice that enhances your life. This mindful approach not only makes the process more enjoyable but also deeply enriches your understanding of your body's responses, leading to more personalized and effective health strategies.

2.4 NUTRITIONAL GUIDELINES TO FOLLOW BEFORE STARTING IF

As you prepare to incorporate intermittent fasting into your lifestyle, laying a solid nutritional foundation is crucial. Think of your body as a garden; just as plants need rich soil to flourish, your body needs a well-balanced diet to thrive, especially during non-fasting periods. This approach ensures that intermittent fasting becomes a positive force in your life, enhancing your overall health rather than depleting it.

A balanced diet is vital, particularly one that is rich in nutrients. For women over 50, the foods you choose to eat during your eating windows significantly impact how your body responds to fasting. It's not just about filling your plate; it's about choosing the right kinds of foods that support hormonal balance, bone health, and muscular function—areas that often need more attention as you age. Foods rich in calcium and vitamin D, such as dairy products or fortified alternatives, are essential for bone health. Meanwhile, lean proteins support muscle repair and growth, whether from animal sources like fish and chicken or plant-based sources like lentils and chickpeas.

Focusing on foods that support hormonal balance is also crucial. Flaxseeds, for instance, are known for their phytoestrogens, which can help manage estrogen levels. Soy products, too, offer benefits in managing menopausal symptoms while providing high-quality protein. Incorporating a variety of fruits and vegetables can help ensure you get a broad spectrum of vitamins and minerals, which are vital for maintaining numerous bodily functions and helping with detoxification processes during fasting periods.

However, there are common nutritional pitfalls that you might encounter, especially when adjusting to a new eating pattern like intermittent fasting. One of the most significant issues is the potential for nutrient deficits. It's easy to under-consume essential nutrients when you're eating less frequently, which is why each meal should be nutrient-dense. Avoiding overly processed foods that offer little nutritional value and focusing on whole foods can significantly enhance the quality of your diet. Foods high in fiber, such as whole grains, fruits, and vegetables, provide essential nutrients and help keep you feeling full, making the fasting periods more straightforward to manage.

Preparing your body for fasting periods is another critical step. Gradually reducing your intake of sugars and refined carbohydrates a few weeks before you begin fasting can ease the transition. High sugar intake can lead to spikes and crashes in blood sugar levels, which might make fasting periods more challenging due to increased hunger and irritability. Instead, increase your hydration. Drinking adequate fluids is crucial, as hydration status can affect both your energy levels and metabolism. Starting your day with a large glass of water and continuing to drink regularly can help manage hunger and maintain energy levels. Additionally, including hydrating foods like cucumbers, celery, and watermelon can further support your hydration levels.

By focusing on a balanced diet that prioritizes nutrient density and hydration, you set the stage for a more effective and enjoyable intermittent fasting experience. This nutritional approach not only supports your body during fasting periods but also enhances your overall health, providing the nutrients needed for energy, recovery, and longevity. As you prepare meals, consider the colors on your plate—aim for a variety of hues, each representing different nutrients that will help your body thrive during and after your fasting periods. Remember, the goal is to nourish your body and spirit, making intermittent fasting a harmonious part of your quest for health and vitality.

2.5 THE IMPORTANCE OF HYDRATION DURING FASTING PERIODS

When we talk about fasting, often the focus is primarily on food—what and when to eat. However, what's equally crucial and sometimes overlooked is hydration. Maintaining adequate hydration, especially during fasting periods, is pivotal in ensuring the fasting process optimizes your body. It's not just about quenching thirst; it's about supporting your body's metabolic functions and aiding in the detoxification processes that are so vital when you're giving your digestive system a break.

Water is a fundamental component of our bodies, involved in every single bodily process, including circulation, digestion, and temperature regulation. When you fast, your body continues to require water to break down fat for energy and to help dispose of the toxins that are released during this process. Additionally, staying hydrated can help curb some of the initial side effects of fasting, such as headaches or dizziness, which can sometimes be exacerbated by dehydration.

Now, how much water should you drink? The general guideline of eight 8-ounce glasses per day is a good starting point, but it's important to remember that everyone's needs are different. During fasting, a good rule of thumb is to listen to your body and drink when thirsty. You might find that you need slightly more water than usual, especially as your body adjusts to your new eating schedule. It's also wise to spread your water intake evenly throughout your eating window and ensure you're well-hydrated before you start your fast. This can help manage hunger and maintain energy levels, making the fasting periods more comfortable.

Recognizing the signs of dehydration is crucial, especially if you're new to fasting. Common symptoms include dry mouth, fatigue, dark urine, and infrequent urination. If you notice these signs, increase your water intake. Remember, symptoms like headaches or lethargy, often dismissed as 'normal' fasting effects, are your body signaling for more fluids.

Let's not forget about electrolytes—minerals in your body that include sodium, potassium, and magnesium. They play vital roles in maintaining fluid balance and are essential for normal function of cells and nerves. When you fast, especially for longer durations, your body loses water and these vital electrolytes. Including a source of electrolytes in your diet can help maintain the balance. Natural sources include coconut water, which is high in potassium, and broth, which provides sodium. If you prefer, electrolyte supplements are available, but they are aimed at those without added sugars or artificial flavorings.

Maintaining hydration and electrolyte balance is not just a matter of health during fasting; it's a practice that enhances the overall effectiveness of your fasting routine. It ensures that your body functions optimally, supports the natural detox processes, and helps you feel better physically and mentally during fasting. So next time you prepare for a fast, remember to give water the attention it deserves—your body will thank you for it.

2.6 MENTAL PREPARATION: BUILDING A RESILIENT MINDSET

When you step into intermittent fasting, you're not just reshaping your eating patterns; you're also embarking on a mental shift that requires resilience, positivity, and an adaptable mindset. Think of it as preparing the soil before you plant seeds. You wouldn't toss seeds onto unprepared ground and hope for the best. Similarly, preparing your mind for the changes intermittent fasting brings is crucial for success.

Cultivating a positive outlook is pivotal. This doesn't mean ignoring the challenges or pretending that difficulties don't exist; rather, it's about acknowledging the hurdles while focusing on the potential benefits and progress. Techniques such as visualizing your goals can be incredibly motivating. Imagine feeling more energetic, healthier, and revitalized. Keeping these images at the forefront of your mind can propel you through moments of doubt or temptation. Additionally, setting small, manageable milestones can help maintain your motivation. Rather than focusing solely on long-term outcomes, celebrate the more minor achievements along the way, like completing your first week of fasting or choosing a healthy meal during your eating window.

Stress, including intermittent fasting, can be a significant barrier to any lifestyle change. It can undermine your efforts by making you reach for comfort foods and affect your body's ability to process those foods efficiently. Managing stress is, therefore, critical to your fasting success. Techniques such as meditation, yoga, and regular physical activity reduce stress and enhance your overall well-being, making you more resilient to the ups and downs of adopting a new eating pattern. Meditation, for instance, doesn't require elaborate setups or excessive time; just a few minutes each day can center your thoughts and calm your mind. Similarly, yoga combines physical movement with breath control and meditation, providing a holistic approach to stress relief. Even simple daily walks can significantly uplift your mood and improve your physical health.

Building a support system can significantly enhance your fasting experience. Just as plants thrive better in a garden with good neighbors, having a supportive community can help you navigate the intermittent fasting path more smoothly. This could be through online forums, local support groups, or even a buddy who embarks on the intermittent fasting journey with you. Sharing experiences, challenges, and successes with others who understand what you're going through creates a sense of camaraderie and mutual support. It's encouraging to hear others' success stories and learn from their experiences, and equally important to have a safe space to express any difficulties and receive constructive feedback.

Finally, preparing for emotional fluctuations is essential. Dietary changes can trigger surprising emotional responses. You might sometimes feel irritable or low, especially as your body adjusts to new eating schedules. Recognizing that these feelings are normal and temporary can help you manage them more effectively. Practicing self-care is crucial. This might involve ensuring you get enough sleep, engaging in relaxing hobbies, or simply allowing yourself time to rest and rejuvenate. Being patient with yourself and acknowledging that adjustments take time can help you maintain a balanced perspective.

Navigating the mental aspects of intermittent fasting is as crucial as managing the dietary components. By fostering a positive mindset, managing stress effectively, building a supportive community, and preparing for emotional ups and downs, you equip yourself with the tools necessary for a successful fasting experience. This preparation supports your current transition and strengthens your overall resilience, enhancing your ability to handle other challenges in life.

As this chapter concludes, remember that mental preparation is not just about making intermittent fasting easier; it's about transforming it into a positive, enriching experience that contributes to your overall growth and well-being. The strategies discussed here lay the groundwork for a resilient mindset that not only navigates the challenges of fasting but also embraces the opportunities it presents for personal development and health improvement.

Looking ahead, the next chapter will build on these foundations, exploring the physical and practical adjustments necessary to integrate intermittent fasting seamlessly into your daily life. By understanding and aligning both mental and physical strategies, you'll be better equipped to enjoy the journey and reap the maximum benefits of your new eating pattern.

INTERMITTENT FASTING METHODS AND SCHEDULES

Imagine you're standing before a buffet of time management options, each dish offering a unique flavor of intermittent fasting. Just as you might choose different meals based on your dietary needs, mood, or occasion, selecting a fasting method is deeply personal, depending on your lifestyle, health, and personal preferences. This chapter serves as your menu, guiding you through various intermittent fasting methods and helping you find the one that resonates best with your life.

3.1 EXPLORING DIFFERENT FASTING WINDOWS: 16/8, 5:2, AND MORE

Overview of Popular Methods

The intermittent fasting landscape is diverse, offering several methods that cater to different lifestyles and health goals. Let's explore three popular methods: 16/8, 5:2, and Eat-Stop-Eat.

The 16/8 method, also known as time-restricted eating, involves fasting for 16 hours each day and eating within an 8-hour window. It's one of the most popular and manageable approaches, especially for those new to fasting. This method is as simple as skipping breakfast and eating your first meal at noon and your last meal by 8 PM.

Then there's the 5:2 method, which involves eating normally five days a week and reducing your calorie intake to about 500-600 calories on the other two non-consecutive days. This method is particularly appealing if you find daily fasting too restrictive and prefer significant calorie reduction a couple of times a week instead.

The Eat-Stop-Eat approach pushes the envelope a bit further, involving a 24-hour fast once or twice a week. Starting from dinner one day and fasting until dinner the next day, this method can be quite challenging but effective for those who seek more pronounced fasting benefits and can manage longer periods without eating.

Choosing the Right Window

Selecting the right fasting method is like choosing the right pair of shoes; it needs to fit well and suit your lifestyle. Consider your daily routine, health status, and how you handle periods without food. If you have a busy morning schedule, the 16/8 method might suit you, allowing you to skip breakfast and focus on your tasks. If you can handle sporadic calorie restriction and prefer less frequent intervention, the 5:2 method might be your match.

It's also important to consider gradual adaptation. Start with the less restrictive method and gradually build your fasting muscle. For instance, begin with the 16/8 method, and as you become more comfortable, experiment with the 5:2 or even the Eat-Stop-Eat method if you're inclined.

Benefits of Each Method

Each fasting method offers distinct benefits. The 16/8 method is particularly flexible, easily fitting into most lifestyles, and is less likely to disrupt social meals or family time. It's also been shown to improve insulin sensitivity, aid weight management, and even extend lifespan.

While the 5:2 method requires more discipline on fasting days, it allows more freedom during the rest of the week. It can significantly reduce calorie intake without the daily commitment, which might be easier for some to maintain in the long term.

Although the most challenging, the Eat-Stop-Eat method can lead to substantial benefits in terms of weight loss and metabolic health. It's a powerful tool for those looking to make considerable changes in their health metrics and can be a test of mental discipline and physical endurance.

Spontaneous meal skipping, a flexible form of intermittent fasting, offers several benefits. It allows individuals to listen to their bodies' natural hunger signals, potentially leading to reduced calorie intake and weight loss. This approach can improve metabolic health by giving the digestive system regular breaks, which may enhance insulin sensitivity and blood sugar control. Additionally, spontaneous meal skipping can simplify meal planning and reduce the stress associated with rigid eating schedules, making it easier to maintain a healthy lifestyle.

Transitioning Between Methods

Transitioning between fasting methods should be handled carefully, akin to acclimating to a new climate. Pay attention to how your body responds to each method. Some may find the 16/8 method a perfect lifelong fit, while others might evolve from 16/8 to 5:2 as their needs and goals change.

Consider your physical response—how do you feel during and after fasting? Monitor your energy levels, mental clarity, and overall well-being. Also, think about your personal schedule—what times of the year or month do you find you have more social engagements or stress? These factors can influence which fasting method fits best at any given time.

Remember, intermittent fasting isn't a one-size-fits-all solution; it's a personal tool that you can tailor to fit your unique health needs and lifestyle. Whether that be adjusting the 16/8 method to 12/12, or increasing the calorie intake on the 5:2 method. IF is flexible; finding a pattern that fits your lifestyle and listening to your body's responses is critical to sustaining this practice without feeling deprived or overly stressed.

Journaling Prompt: Reflective Exercise

To help you decide which intermittent fasting method might suit you best, take a moment to reflect on your typical day. How does your current schedule align with potential eating and fasting windows? What are your personal and professional commitments, and how might they affect your ability to maintain a fasting schedule? Write down your thoughts and consider how each method might fit into your lifestyle. This exercise can provide clarity and help you make a practical and exciting choice, setting you up for success in your intermittent fasting adventure.

In this chapter, we've navigated the varied landscape of intermittent fasting methods, each with its unique rhythm and requirements. As you consider your options, remember that the best approach is one that feels sustainable and resonant with your lifestyle. Whether you choose the flexibility of the 16/8 method, the periodic commitment of the 5:2 method, or the intensity of the Eat-Stop-Eat approach, the key is to listen to your body and choose a path that supports your health goals and daily life.

3.2 TIME-RESTRICTED EATING: A DAY IN THE LIFE

Visualize a fresh Wednesday dawn, the early sunlight beginning to streak across the sky. As a dynamic woman over 50, you're poised to embark on a day enriched by the sharpness and vitality provided by your 16/8 intermittent fasting routine. Your designated eating period is from 12 noon to 8 PM, seamlessly integrating with your daily routine of professional duties, personal endeavors, and family interactions.

You start your day at 6 AM, refreshed and ready after a good night's sleep. Breakfast isn't on your mind just yet despite the early hour because your body is now attuned to this eating schedule. Instead, you hydrate with a tall glass of water and perhaps a warm cup of herbal tea. Hydration in the morning is crucial; it kickstarts your metabolism and helps maintain your cognitive function. You then lace up for a brisk walk. This morning exercise isn't just about physical health; it's a cherished quiet time, allowing you to collect your thoughts and plan your day.

By 9 AM, you're diving into work. The focus here is incredible—something you've noticed has significantly improved since starting intermittent fasting. Mid-morning, you might feel a slight hunger pang; it's nothing a second glass of water or another cup of tea can't handle. This is also an excellent time to take supplements that don't require food to be effective, ensuring you're supporting your body's nutrient needs.

Lunch at noon is a joyful affair; it's not just your first meal of the day but a break, to really enjoy what you're eating. You opt for a balanced meal: perhaps a vibrant salad with leafy greens, chickpeas for protein, a good portion of avocados for healthy fats, and a sprinkling of nuts for crunch. This satisfies your hunger and ensures you're packed with nutrients to power through the afternoon.

Post-lunch, your afternoon is a blend of work and personal chores, all performed with a steady energy level—no post-lunch slump in sight, thanks to your well-balanced meal. As the end of your eating window approaches, dinner around 7:30 PM consists of grilled salmon, a side of roasted vegetables, and quinoa—foods that are not only delicious but are also slowly digested, which will help sustain your energy levels through the fasting period.

Throughout your eating window, you continue to hydrate, helping your digestion and maintaining hydration. Your routine might differ slightly if you're an early riser or tend to stay up later. For early risers, shifting the eating window earlier, say from 10 AM to 6 PM, ensures you're not going to bed on a full stomach, which can disrupt sleep. For night owls, shifting the window to later in the day, from 2 PM to 10 PM, might suit your lifestyle better, allowing you to have a social dinner or late work meetings, without breaking your fast.

Adapting your fasting schedule to fit your sleep pattern and daily routine is critical to maintaining energy and enthusiasm for intermittent fasting. It's this flexibility that makes time-restricted eating a sustainable choice, not just for those looking to manage their weight but for anyone seeking a structured yet adaptable way to improve overall health. As your day winds down, you prepare for the next fast, feeling satisfied and in tune with your body's rhythm, ready to embrace the quiet of the evening and the restorative power of sleep, knowing tomorrow is another opportunity to nourish, thrive, and enjoy every moment.

3.3 THE 5:2 METHOD: DETAILED WEEKLY PLAN

Imagine reshaping your eating habits not by subtracting but by strategically adjusting when and how much you eat on just two days a week. This is the essence of the 5:2 method of intermittent fasting, which integrates beautifully into the lives of women over 50 who are balancing the dynamics of work, life, and ever-changing physical needs. Let's walk through a sample weekly plan that not only illustrates the practical application of the 5:2 method but also ensures that you're nourished, satisfied, and ready to embrace this moderate approach to fasting.

Consider beginning your week on Monday with a typical eating day, where "normal" reflects a balanced diet rich in vegetables, whole grains, lean proteins, and healthy fats. This sets a positive tone for the week, providing you with ample energy and nutrients. Tuesday then becomes your first reduced-calorie day. On this day, aim for meals that are high in nutrients but lower in calories. A breakfast might not be on the menu, giving you an extended overnight fast. For lunch, consider a broth-based soup with plenty of vegetables and some lean protein, such as chicken or tofu. Dinner could be a salad dressed with lemon juice and a small drizzle of olive oil, topped with a portion of grilled fish or a handful of chickpeas. The key here is to focus on high-volume, low-calorie foods that fill you up without excessive calories.

Wednesday and Thursday are regular eating days again, allowing more flexibility. Enjoy nourishing meals that emphasize whole foods, and perhaps treat yourself to a favorite dish that you look forward to, maintaining a joyful relationship with food. Friday, the second low-calorie day, mirrors Tuesday but with an intention to vary the menu to keep things interesting and nutritionally diverse. Maybe you start your day with a green smoothie packed with spinach, a small banana, and a scoop of protein powder. Dinner could be stir-fried veggies with just a touch of soy sauce and sesame oil, served over a modest scoop of cauliflower rice.

The weekend is free from fasting constraints, allowing you to socialize, relax, and enjoy meals with family or friends. This rhythm helps manage your caloric intake over the week and aligns with typical social patterns, where weekends might offer more culinary temptations.

Meal Planning for Fast Days

Planning your meals on fast days is crucial to ensure you remain energized and satisfied. Choose foods rich in fiber and protein, as these nutrients help slow digestion and can reduce hunger pangs. Soups and salads are excellent choices as they can be filling while still being low in calories. Including a good variety of vegetables helps ensure you get a range of nutrients that might otherwise be limited due to reduced food intake. Planning ahead can prevent the temptation to reach for convenient, higher-calorie foods that might sabotage your fasting efforts.

Balancing Nutrient Intake

Over the week, it's essential to maintain a balance between your macronutrients (proteins, fats, carbohydrates) and micronutrients (vitamins and minerals). On regular eating days, ensure your meals are varied and cover all food groups to compensate for the more restrictive days. Including foods like berries, nuts, seeds, and leafy greens across the week will help boost your intake of vitamins, minerals, and antioxidants, supporting overall health and compensating for the lower intake on fast days.

Monitoring Body Response

Adopting and adapting to the 5:2 method requires attentive listening to your body's physical and emotional responses. It's beneficial to keep a journal to note how you feel on fast days compared to regular eating days. Are you unusually tired? Do you feel irritable? How is your hunger level? Adjustments might be necessary based on your observations. For example, if you're too fatigued on fast days, it might help to slightly increase your calorie intake or adjust the timing of your meals. This mindful approach to fasting helps optimize the method to work best for you and ensures that you maintain it comfortably and beneficially in the long run.

By tailoring the 5:2 method to fit your needs and lifestyle and carefully planning and monitoring your food intake and responses, you create a fasting rhythm that feels less like a diet and more like a sustainable part of a healthy, vibrant lifestyle. As you continue to explore and adjust, remember that this method is flexible and designed to adapt to your life's rhythms and nutritional needs.

3.4 THE EAT STOP EAT METHOD: DETAILED WEEKLY PLAN

Envisage reshaping your eating habits not by subtracting, but by strategically adjusting when you eat for 24 hours, once or twice a week. This is the essence of the Eat Stop Eat method of intermittent fasting, which integrates beautifully into the lives of women over 50 who are balancing the dynamics of work, life, and ever-changing physical needs. Let's walk through a sample weekly plan that not only illustrates the practical application of the Eat Stop Eat method but also ensures that you are nourished, satisfied, and ready to embrace this moderate approach to fasting.

Consider beginning your week on Monday with a typical eating day, where "normal" reflects a balanced diet rich in vegetables, whole grains, lean proteins, and healthy fats. This sets a positive tone for the week, providing you with ample energy and nutrients. On Tuesday, you might decide to start your first 24-hour fast after dinner, so you would eat dinner at around 7 PM and then not eat again until 7 PM on Wednesday. During fasting, focus on staying hydrated with water, herbal tea, or black coffee.

Wednesday evening marks the end of your fast. Break your fast with a nutritious, balanced meal that's easy to digest, such as a mixed greens salad with roasted sweet potatoes, chickpeas, avocado, and grilled chicken. Thursday and Friday are regular eating days again, allowing more flexibility. Enjoy nourishing meals that emphasize whole foods, and perhaps treat yourself to a favorite dish that you look forward to, maintaining a joyful relationship with food.

Saturday becomes your second 24-hour fasting day, starting after breakfast or lunch, depending on your schedule and preference. For example, you might finish lunch at 1 PM and fast until 1 PM on Sunday. During the fasting period, again focus on hydration and perhaps light physical activity, like a gentle walk, to stay active without overexerting yourself.

Sunday afternoons and evenings are free from fasting constraints, allowing you to socialize, relax, and enjoy meals with family or friends.

Meal Planning for Fast Days

Planning your meals on regular eating days is crucial to ensure you remain energized and satisfied. Choose foods rich in fiber and protein, as these nutrients help slow digestion and can reduce hunger pangs. Soups and salads are excellent choices as they can be filling while still being low in calories. Including a good variety of vegetables helps ensure you get a range of nutrients that might otherwise be limited due to reduced food intake.

Balancing Nutrient Intake

Over the week, it's essential to maintain a balance between your macronutrients (proteins, fats, carbohydrates) and micronutrients (vitamins and minerals). On regular eating days, ensure your meals are varied and cover all food groups to compensate for the more restrictive days. Including foods like berries, nuts, seeds, and leafy greens across the week will help boost your intake of vitamins, minerals, and antioxidants, supporting overall health and compensating for the lower intake on fast days.

Monitoring Body Response

Adopting and adapting to the Eat Stop Eat method requires attentive listening to your body's physical and emotional responses. Keeping a journal to note how you feel on fasting days compared to regular eating days is beneficial. Are you unusually tired? Do you feel irritable? How is your hunger level? Adjustments might be necessary based on your observations. For example, if you're too tired on fasting days, it might help to slightly increase your calorie intake on non-fasting days or adjust the timing of your meals. This mindful approach to fasting helps optimize the method to work best for you and ensures that you maintain it comfortably and beneficially in the long run.

By tailoring the Eat Stop Eat method to fit your needs and lifestyle and carefully planning and monitoring your food intake and responses, you create a fasting rhythm that feels less like a diet and more like a sustainable part of a healthy, vibrant lifestyle. As you continue to explore and adjust, remember that this method is flexible and designed to adapt to your life's rhythms and nutritional needs.

3.5 PROS AND CONS OF SPONTANEOUS MEAL SKIPPING

In the landscape of intermittent fasting, spontaneous meal skipping is akin to an impromptu dance; it's flexible, adaptable, and allows you to move with the rhythms of your day-to-day life without strict scheduling. This method involves skipping meals on an as-needed basis rather than following a predetermined fasting schedule. For instance, if you wake up one morning and you're not particularly hungry, you might decide to skip breakfast and wait until lunch to eat. This approach is noticeably different from structured fasting plans that set specific times for eating and fasting.

The beauty of spontaneous meal skipping lies in its inherent flexibility. This method is incredibly accommodating for those with fluctuating schedules—perhaps your days are filled with varying work hours, social commitments, or family responsibilities that make adhering to a strict eating schedule challenging. Spontaneous meal skipping can easily become part of your lifestyle, allowing you to adjust your food intake based on actual hunger signals rather than the clock. This can lead to a more intuitive relationship with food, where you eat in response to your body's needs rather than external time cues.

However, this flexibility comes with potential challenges, particularly concerning nutritional balance. The ad-hoc nature of spontaneous meal skipping means you might miss out on essential nutrients if not carefully managed. Without the structure of planned meals, it's easy to end up either under-eating, which could lead to nutrient deficiencies, or overeating during other meals, which can counteract the benefits of skipping a meal in the first place. Ensuring a balanced intake of proteins, fats, carbohydrates, vitamins, and minerals is crucial, especially for women over 50 who might already be navigating through complex dietary needs due to menopause and metabolic changes.

Adopting best practices for spontaneous meal skipping is critical to navigating these waters successfully. Here are a few tips to ensure that you maintain a healthy balance:

1. **Listen to Your Body:** Learn to recognize true hunger cues and differentiate them from habits or emotional eating. If you decide to skip a meal, assess your energy levels and hunger throughout the day and adjust your subsequent meals to compensate nutritionally.
2. **Plan Nutrient-Dense Meals:** When you do eat, focus on nutrient-dense foods. Include a variety of vegetables, lean proteins, healthy fats, and whole grains that can provide a broad spectrum of nutrients. This ensures that even if you eat less frequently, you still receive the necessary vitamins and minerals your body needs.
3. **Hydrate Adequately:** Hydration is often overlooked when meals are skipped. Ensure you drink plenty of water throughout the day, as fluids are vital for maintaining bodily functions and can help manage hunger.

4. **Monitor Your Health:** Monitor your overall health and energy. If you feel fatigued or irritable or notice any other concerning symptoms, reassess your meal-skipping habits to ensure they're not adversely affecting your health.

By integrating these practices, spontaneous meal skipping can indeed be a practical and flexible approach to intermittent fasting that aligns with the unpredictable nature of daily life. It encourages a form of dietary freedom and body attunement that many structured plans do not, fostering a deeper connection with your body's natural hunger signals and needs. As you continue to navigate this method, remember that the goal is to find a balance that feels nourishing and sustainable, allowing you to enjoy the myriad activities and joys of your life without feeling constrained by your dietary choices.

3.6 CUSTOMIZING YOUR FASTING PLAN: ADJUSTMENTS FOR ENERGY AND HUNGER

When embarking on an intermittent fasting plan, one size certainly does not fit all, especially for women over 50, who may experience significant fluctuations in energy due to hormonal changes and other physiological adjustments. It's crucial to recognize that your energy needs are unique and may vary from day to day. Adjusting your fasting plan to accommodate these changes can make the difference between a struggle and a sustainable lifestyle shift.

Start by closely monitoring how different fasting windows affect your energy levels. For instance, if you find that a longer fasting period leaves you feeling lethargic or irritable, it might be a sign that your body prefers shorter fasting windows or needs a slight adjustment in meal timing or composition. It's helpful to keep a detailed diary of how you feel during different fasting periods. Note any changes in your energy levels, mood, and overall well-being. This record can be invaluable as you tweak your fasting schedule to better fit your body's needs.

Additionally, consider the nature of your daily activities. If your days are filled with demanding physical tasks or require high mental focus, you might need to schedule your eating windows to ensure you are well-fueled during these times. For some, having a hearty, nutrient-rich meal before a challenging day can help maintain high energy levels. In contrast, others might find that eating after a strenuous activity improves recovery and satisfaction.

Managing Hunger During Fasting Periods

Managing hunger is another critical aspect of customizing your fasting plan. It's natural to feel hungry during fasting periods, especially in the beginning. However, managing this hunger can impact your overall experience and success with intermittent fasting. One effective strategy is to focus on high-fiber and protein-rich foods during your eating windows. Foods like legumes, whole grains, lean proteins, and vegetables can increase satiety and prevent extreme hunger during fasting periods. These nutrients have a slower digestion rate, which helps in gradually releasing energy, keeping you fuller for longer.

Another helpful approach is to incorporate healthy fats into your meals. Foods rich in omega-3 fatty acids, such as fish, nuts, and seeds, support your heart health and increase fullness. Including a variety of these foods can make your meals both satisfying and nourishing, helping you manage hunger more effectively throughout your fasting periods.

Listening to Your Body's Feedback

Listening to your body's feedback is paramount in adjusting your fasting plan effectively. This means paying attention to your hunger and energy levels and other signals your body might be sending you. Are you sleeping well? Do you feel hydrated? How are your concentration and overall mood? These clues can help you fine-tune your fasting schedule to better suit your health needs.

For example, if you notice that you're feeling unusually fatigued or unable to focus well during certain times of your fasting period, it might be necessary to adjust your nutrient intake during your eating windows or slightly alter your fasting hours. It's important to approach these adjustments with a willingness to experiment and find what truly works for your body.

Experimentation and Patience

Finally, embracing experimentation and patience is essential as you find the fasting rhythm that works best for you. The effects of intermittent fasting can vary widely among individuals, and what works wonderfully for one person might not be ideal for another. It's okay to try different fasting methods, adjust your eating windows, and experiment with meal compositions until you find a balance that feels right.

Remember, finding the perfect fasting plan is a journey that might take time. Be patient with yourself and allow your body to gradually adapt to the changes. Celebrate small victories along the way, and don't hesitate to make adjustments as your lifestyle and body's needs evolve. This flexible, patient approach not only makes intermittent fasting more enjoyable but also enhances its sustainability in the long run, helping you maintain your health and vitality well beyond your fifties

3.7 COMBINING INTERMITTENT FASTING WITH OTHER DIETS

When you think about blending intermittent fasting with other diet plans, imagine it as pairing fine wine with the right kind of cheese; each enhances the flavor of the other, creating a delightful synergy that elevates your dining experience. Similarly, combining intermittent fasting with specific diets like ketogenic, Mediterranean, or plant-based diets can significantly enhance health benefits, each complementing the other in ways that can lead to a richer, more fulfilling lifestyle change.

Starting with the ketogenic diet, which is high in fats and low in carbohydrates, it naturally complements intermittent fasting. When you fast, your body begins to deplete its glucose reserves and starts to burn fat for energy, a state known as ketosis. By adopting a ketogenic diet, you're essentially priming your body to enter this fat-burning state more efficiently, even outside of fasting periods. This can accelerate weight loss and improve your lipid profiles, including cholesterol and triglycerides. It's a powerful combination for those particularly focused on heart health and metabolic improvements.

Switching to the Mediterranean diet, which is rich in vegetables, fruits, nuts, seeds, legumes, whole grains, and olive oil and includes moderate amounts of fish and poultry, it's celebrated for its anti-inflammatory properties. When combined with intermittent fasting, the effects can be particularly beneficial. Fasting itself has been shown to reduce markers of inflammation, so when paired with a diet known for its anti-inflammatory effects, you can significantly enhance your body's overall inflammatory response. This is particularly important for women over 50, as inflammation can contribute to chronic diseases prevalent in this age group, such as heart disease, diabetes, and arthritis.

However, while the benefits are compelling, there are essential considerations and cautions. Nutritional balance is paramount. For instance, while the ketogenic diet can be effective in accelerating fat loss, it's also high in fats, and care must be taken to ensure these are primarily healthy fats. Additionally, because it restricts carbohydrates, there's a risk of nutrient deficiency if not correctly managed. Similarly, while the Mediterranean diet is diverse in its food choices, its effectiveness can be diminished if the proportion of processed foods is too high or if portion control is ignored.

Let's consider some anecdotes to bring these concepts to life. Take the case of Linda, a 58-year-old who combined intermittent fasting with the ketogenic diet. She not only lost weight but also saw a significant drop in her cholesterol levels. Linda found that her energy levels were sustained better throughout the day, and she felt less of the mid-afternoon slump she typically experienced. Then there's Maria, who adopted the Mediterranean diet alongside her intermittent fasting routine. She noticed not only a decrease in her weight but also a significant reduction in joint pain and stiffness, which she attributed to the anti-inflammatory benefits of her combined dietary approach.

These stories underscore the transformative potential of combining intermittent fasting with specific diets tailored to individual health needs and lifestyle preferences. As you consider integrating these methods into your life, it's crucial to consult with healthcare providers to tailor the approach to your specific health conditions and nutritional needs. This ensures that you maintain a balanced and healthful diet while reaping the maximum benefits of your chosen dietary synergy.

Combining intermittent fasting with other dietary approaches like ketogenic, Mediterranean, or plant-based diets can significantly enhance health benefits. This chapter has explored how each diet complements intermittent fasting, helping to improve lipid profiles, enhance anti-inflammatory effects, and ensure a broader range of nutrients. As we move forward, keep in mind the importance of customization to your personal health needs and preferences, ensuring that your dietary plan is not only effective but also enjoyable and sustainable.

NUTRITION AND MEAL PLANNING

Imagine you're navigating a bustling market, each stall brimming with nutrient-rich foods that promise to nourish your body and enhance your fasting experience. As you meander through the colorful arrays of fresh produce, you're not just shopping; you're crafting a dietary strategy that supports your vibrant lifestyle over 50. This chapter is your guide through the nutrition marketplace, focusing specifically on the essential nutrients and supplements that can bolster your health as you embrace intermittent fasting.

4.1 ESSENTIAL NUTRIENTS AND SUPPLEMENTS FOR WOMEN OVER 50

Navigating nutrition in your fifties and beyond can sometimes feel like trying to solve a complex puzzle. Your body's needs have shifted, and suddenly, you're not just eating to satisfy hunger but strategically to bolster bone density, enhance heart health, and maintain energy levels. Let's break down the vital nutrients for women over 50 and how you can ensure you're getting enough of them through diet and supplements.

Identifying Key Nutrients

Firstly, calcium is paramount for maintaining bone density, which becomes crucial as you age and your risk of osteoporosis increases. The daily recommended intake is about 1,200 mg for women over 50. Dairy products like milk, cheese, and yogurt are rich in calcium, but if you're dairy-free, you can turn to fortified plant milks, leafy greens, and almonds.

Vitamin D is essential for calcium absorption, and it plays a significant role in immune function and fighting inflammation. While sunlight is a primary source, many people don't get enough sun exposure, especially in the winter months. Foods like salmon, fortified cereals, and eggs provide Vitamin D, but supplementation is often necessary to reach the recommended daily intake of 600 to 800 IU.

Omega-3 fatty acids are your heart's best friend. They help lower blood pressure, reduce triglycerides, and even decrease the risk of stroke—vital considerations for women over 50. Fatty fish like salmon and mackerel are excellent sources, but flaxseeds and walnuts are great alternatives for those who don't eat fish.

Role of Supplements

While aiming to get most of your nutrients from food is ideal, supplements play a crucial role in filling any gaps, especially for nutrients that are hard to obtain in sufficient quantities through diet alone. Vitamin B12, crucial for nerve function and DNA and red blood cell production, is one such nutrient. It's predominantly found in animal products, and absorbing enough B12 from diet alone can be challenging due to decreased stomach acid production with age. A B12 supplement can be particularly beneficial.

Magnesium is another nutrient vital for bone health, regulating muscle and nerve function, and maintaining blood sugar levels. While it's present in various foods, including whole grains, nuts, and greens, supplementing with magnesium can ensure you meet your daily needs, which is particularly important for those who are managing type 2 diabetes or cardiovascular health.

Interactions with Fasting

Integrating supplements into your intermittent fasting schedule requires careful timing to maximize absorption and effectiveness. Fat-soluble vitamins like Vitamins D, E, A, and K should be taken during your eating window as they require fat from your meals for optimal absorption. However, water-soluble vitamins like Vitamin C and most B vitamins can be taken outside your eating window as they do not need to be taken with food and can be absorbed directly through the intestinal tract.

Customized Supplement Plans

Consulting with a healthcare provider to tailor your supplement plan is key. They can offer guidance based on a comprehensive evaluation of your health needs, dietary intake, and fasting schedule. This personalized approach ensures that you supplement wisely, enhancing your diet without causing imbalances or over-supplementation, which can be just as harmful as a deficiency.

Interactive Element: Journaling Prompt

Keep a food and supplement diary for a week to better understand your nutritional intake and supplement needs. Record everything you eat and any supplements you take, noting how you feel physically and mentally. Review this diary with your healthcare provider to identify any gaps or adjustments needed to optimize your nutrition and overall health.

In this thorough exploration of essential nutrients and supplements for women over 50, we've delved into why these dietary components are crucial for maintaining health and vitality during and beyond your fasting journey. By understanding how to effectively incorporate these nutrients into your diet, either through food or supplements, and recognizing the importance of timing concerning your fasting schedule, you equip yourself with the knowledge to make informed choices that bolster your health, enabling you to thrive in this vibrant chapter of your life.

4.2 BUILDING A MENOPAUSE-FRIENDLY MEAL PLAN

Navigating through menopause can sometimes feel like you're trying to solve a complex puzzle where the pieces are your fluctuating hormones, changing energy levels, and a body that doesn't always respond as predictably as it used to. Crafting a menopause-friendly meal plan means more than just filling your plate; it's about crafting a strategy that addresses these changes head-on, helping you manage common menopausal symptoms like hot flushes, weight gain, and mood swings. The key is focusing on dietary strategies that support hormonal balance and stabilize your metabolism through these transitions.

Let's start with the reality of hot flushes and mood swings—frequent and sometimes frustrating visitors during menopause.

Adjusting your diet to manage these symptoms can be incredibly effective. Incorporating foods rich in phytoestrogens, such as flaxseeds and soy products, is a natural approach to help balance your hormone levels. Phytoestrogens are plant-derived compounds that mimic the effects of estrogen in the body, potentially easing the severity of hot flashes and smoothing out mood fluctuations. Flaxseeds can be an excellent addition to your morning smoothie or sprinkled over a salad while incorporating tofu or tempeh into your meals can offer a hearty, phytoestrogen-rich protein source.

Weight management becomes a bit trickier during menopause due to the metabolic slowdown that often accompanies hormonal changes. Integrating low-glycemic index foods into your diet can be a game-changer here. Foods with a low glycemic index, such as whole grains, legumes, and most fruits and vegetables, have a slower impact on your blood sugar levels. This slower absorption helps prevent the spikes and crashes that can lead to increased hunger and subsequent weight gain. For example, starting your day with a bowl of steel-cut oats topped with berries offers a filling, low-glycemic breakfast that keeps your energy levels steady throughout the morning. For lunch, a quinoa and chickpea salad dressed with olive oil and lemon juice can provide a satisfying and nutritious option that won't send your blood sugar soaring.

Meal timing and frequency also play crucial roles in managing menopausal symptoms effectively. Aligning your meal times with your natural energy fluctuations can help you feel more balanced throughout the day. You might find that eating a substantial, protein-rich breakfast helps stabilize your mood and energy levels, reducing the intensity of hot flushes throughout the day. Conversely, a light dinner can prevent sleep disturbances often exacerbated by heavy evening meals. Maintaining a consistent eating schedule is also beneficial to help regulate your metabolism, which can become less predictable during menopause. Eating your meals at similar times each day can help your body adapt to the changes it's undergoing, making it easier to manage symptoms like weight gain and mood swings.

Crafting a menopause-friendly meal plan isn't just about choosing the right foods; it's about creating a dietary pattern that supports your body's changing needs. By focusing on phytoestrogens to balance hormones, incorporating low-glycemic foods to manage weight, and aligning meal timing with your body's natural rhythms, you can navigate the challenges of menopause with confidence and comfort. Remember, the goal is to nourish your body and spirit, embracing this phase of life with vitality and grace.

4.3 EASY AND NUTRITIONAL RECIPES FOR NON-FASTING DAYS

When those non-fasting days roll around, it's like a culinary canvas waiting to be painted with vibrant, nutrient-dense foods that satisfy your taste buds and nourish your body deeply. Imagine dishes that are as delightful to your palate as they are beneficial to your health, tailored specifically to support your well-being on days when you aren't fasting. Let's explore some recipes and cooking methods designed to optimize nutrition and enjoyment without adding undue complexity to your meal preparation.

One of the joys of non-fasting days is the opportunity to indulge in a little more culinary creativity. A fantastic start could be a hearty but healthy breakfast of savory oat pancakes. Combine rolled oats, a couple of whisked eggs, chopped spinach, a handful of grated cheese, and a pinch of salt and pepper. Cook these in a non-stick pan with a drop of olive oil until they're golden and firm. These pancakes pack a punch of fiber, protein, and iron while being a delightful twist on a breakfast classic. For lunch, why not try a quinoa and black bean salad? Cooked quinoa, black beans, cherry tomatoes, diced peppers, and corn, dressed with lime juice, olive oil, and a sprinkle of cumin, make for a refreshing, filling meal that's perfect for replenishing your energy stores.

Dinner could be a simple grilled salmon with a side of steamed broccoli and sweet potatoes. Salmon is a fantastic source of omega-3 fatty acids, essential for heart health and cognitive function. At the same time, sweet potatoes provide a rich source of beta-carotene, vital for maintaining healthy skin and eye health. Steaming the broccoli preserves its vitamin C and sulforaphane content, nutrients essential for immune support and detoxification. Finish the day with a dessert of Greek yogurt topped with a mix of berries and a drizzle of honey to boost probiotics, fiber, and antioxidants.

Cooking Methods

The way you cook your food can significantly impact its nutritional content. Steaming is one of the most effective methods to preserve the integrity of your ingredients. It keeps the vegetables vibrant and crunchy, retaining more vitamins and minerals than many other cooking methods. Conversely, grilling can bring out the natural flavors in proteins like fish and chicken without needing much oil or fat. Slow cooking is another excellent option, especially for legumes and stews. It allows herbs and spices to infuse beautifully, creating tasty and tender dishes, and keeping the nutritional profile intact.

Ingredient Swaps

Small tweaks to your favorite recipes' ingredients can substantially enhance their nutritional value. For instance, swapping out white rice for cauliflower rice in your dishes can lower the glycemic index, helping to control blood sugar levels more effectively. Instead of using heavy cream in recipes, try using coconut milk or Greek yogurt to reduce saturated fat while still achieving a creamy texture. These simple swaps help maintain a healthy weight and ensure you're getting a broader range of nutrients in your diet.

Portion Control

It's easy to overindulge on non-fasting days, but maintaining control over your portion sizes is crucial to avoid undoing the benefits of your fasting days. Using smaller plates is a practical trick to help control portions without feeling deprived. Visual cues can also be helpful; for example, a portion of cooked meat should be about the size of a deck of cards, and a serving of grains should fit in the palm of your hand. Being mindful of portion sizes helps maintain a balanced calorie intake and supports sustained weight management, ensuring that you enjoy your meals while keeping your health goals on track.

Through these recipes and tips, you can fully enjoy non-fasting days, ensuring each meal is not only a delight to eat but also a step towards maintaining your health and vitality. Each dish brings a blend of essential nutrients and flavors designed to make your meal times both nourishing and enjoyable. As you integrate these recipes and cooking tips into your routine, you'll find that eating well on non-fasting days becomes a natural, joyful extension of your commitment to a healthier lifestyle.

4.4 SMART SNACKING: WHAT TO EAT DURING YOUR EATING WINDOW

When we talk about maintaining a balanced diet during intermittent fasting, it's not just about the meals; it's also about the snacks that bridge these meals. Think of them as your nutritional pit stops—carefully chosen to fuel your body and mind until your next meal. Snacking smartly during your eating window can significantly affect how you sustain energy, manage hunger, and maintain an overall sense of well-being. It's not just about curbing hunger; it's about making strategic choices that enhance your health.

Choosing Nutrient-Dense Snacks

The importance of selecting snacks that are rich in nutrients—proteins, fiber, and healthy fats—cannot be overstated. These nutrients are crucial in prolonging satiety, stabilizing blood sugar levels, and providing sustained energy. Let's take almonds, for instance. A small handful can be a powerhouse of energy, offering a good mix of protein, fiber, and heart-healthy fats that help keep you feeling full longer. Similarly, a Greek yogurt parfait with a layer of mixed berries and a sprinkle of chia seeds can not only satisfy your taste buds but also provide a rich source of protein, antioxidants, and fiber.

Incorporating such nutrient-dense snacks into your diet doesn't just stave off hunger; it also supports your metabolic health, which is especially crucial in managing the natural metabolic slowdown that can occur after 50. Each snack is an opportunity to feed your body something beneficial, so think of your snacks as mini-meals contributing to your overall nutritional goals.

Snack Timing

Timing your snacks can be just as important as what you eat. Integrating them strategically into your eating window can help maintain energy levels and prevent you from overeating at meal times. A mid-morning snack, for instance, can keep your metabolism active and prevent the common energy dip that may occur midday. A good rule of thumb is to have a snack a couple of hours after a main meal and/or a few hours before the next. This timing helps manage your hunger levels throughout the day, making it less likely that you'll overindulge during your main meals.

For example, if you have lunch at noon and dinner around 7 PM, having a snack around 3 PM can help maintain your energy levels throughout the afternoon. This snack could be something as simple as an apple with a handful of walnuts or a small bowl of mixed vegetables with hummus. These snacks balance carbohydrates, protein, and fats, keeping your energy levels steady and your hunger in check.

Mindful Snacking Tips

Mindful eating is a practice that can transform your relationship with food. It involves paying full attention to the experience of eating and drinking, both inside and outside the body. Pay attention to your food's colors, smells, textures, and flavors; listen to your body's hunger and fullness signals; and notice how different foods affect your emotions and energy levels.

One way to practice mindful snacking is to sit down with your snack, free from distractions like TV or smartphones. This allows you to fully engage with the act of eating and enjoy each bite. It's about quality over quantity, savoring the snack slowly which can lead to greater satisfaction and less likelihood of overeating.

By embracing smart snacking habits—choosing nutrient-dense foods, timing them wisely during your eating window, exploring healthy and quick recipes, and eating mindfully—you enhance your intermittent fasting experience. These snacks become more than just fillers; they are pivotal elements of your diet that contribute to sustained energy, stable blood sugar levels, and overall metabolic health, making every snack a step towards a healthier you.

4.5 PREPARING MEALS FOR ONE: TIPS AND TRICKS

Cooking for one can often seem like a daunting task, especially after a certain age when you're trying to balance health, taste, and convenience. While relying on pre-packaged meals or repetitive dishes might be tempting, there are plenty of strategies to keep your meals fresh, enjoyable, and aligned with your nutritional needs. Let's explore some handy tips and tricks that make cooking for one both simple and pleasurable without sacrificing the quality or variety of your meals.

Efficient Cooking Strategies

One effective strategy to manage meal preparation is batch cooking. This doesn't mean you have to eat the same meal every day; instead, it involves preparing and cooking components of meals in bulk. For instance, you might roast a large tray of mixed vegetables at the start of the week, cook a big pot of quinoa, or grill several chicken breasts. These can then be mixed and matched to create different meals throughout the week, saving you time while ensuring you eat well. Proper storage is critical here—

dividing these cooked foods into portion-sized containers and storing them in the fridge or freezer not only preserves their freshness but also makes it easy to assemble a meal in no time.

Another great strategy is to utilize one-pot dishes, which minimize cleanup and can be easily scaled down for single servings. Soups, stews, and casseroles are all excellent for this kind of cooking. They not only allow for the richness of flavors to develop but are also perfect for incorporating a variety of nutrients into a single dish. Moreover, they usually taste even better the next day, making them ideal for subsequent meals.

Using Leftovers Creatively

Leftovers are inevitable, especially when cooking for one, but they offer a creative challenge that can spice up your meal routine. Transforming leftovers into a new meal is an enjoyable and efficient way to reduce waste while keeping your diet diverse. For example, last night's roasted chicken can become today's chicken salad wrap or a leftover vegetable stir-fry can be mixed with beaten eggs to make a hearty frittata. Even something as simple as old bread can be turned into croutons for a salad or breadcrumbs for coating fish. Viewing leftovers as a base for new culinary creations can make your meals more exciting and enjoyable.

Single-Serving Recipe Ideas

Crafting recipes that cater specifically to single servings can be a delightful exploration. Here are a couple of easy recipes designed just for you:

Stuffed Bell Pepper: Take a large bell pepper, cut off the top, and remove the seeds. Fill it with a mixture of cooked quinoa, black beans, corn, chopped tomatoes, and spices. Top with a sprinkle of cheese and bake in the oven until the pepper is tender and the cheese is bubbly. This meal is easy to prepare and packs a nutritional punch with fiber, protein, and vitamins.

Shrimp and Asparagus Stir Fry: In a pan, sauté a handful of shrimp and asparagus with garlic and a splash of soy sauce. Serve it over a small portion of brown rice for a balanced meal with protein, fiber, and essential nutrients, all tailored to fill you without leftovers.

Shopping Smart

When shopping for one, buying certain items in bulk — think grains, nuts, and frozen goods, which have a long shelf life and can be used in various meals is smart. For fresh produce, buy smaller amounts more frequently to ensure freshness and reduce waste. Many stores sell pre-portioned packets of vegetables, meats, and dairy, which can be more practical for single servings. Another tip is choosing versatile ingredients that can be used in multiple recipes throughout the week, reducing the number of items you need to buy and helping you use up everything you purchase.

By embracing these strategies, meal preparation can become a less daunting and more enjoyable part of your day. It allows you to nourish your body with exactly what it needs, respecting both your health requirements and your palate, without leaving you with a mountain of leftovers or the monotony of the same meal every day. Whether you're batch cooking for efficiency, transforming leftovers with a dash of creativity, or whipping up quick single-serving dishes, these tips ensure that your meals are as delightful to prepare as they are to eat.

4.6 INTEGRATING FAMILY MEALS WITH YOUR IF SCHEDULE

Navigating your intermittent fasting schedule while ensuring family meals remain a source of joy and nutrition can feel like orchestrating a well-tuned symphony. It's about finding the right balance and ensuring your dietary rhythm harmonizes with your family's nutritional needs and preferences. This doesn't mean preparing separate meals for yourself and your loved ones; instead, it involves smart, inclusive meal planning that everyone at the table can enjoy.

The key to successful family meals lies in creating flexible dishes that can be easily adapted to suit both your fasting schedule and your family's nutritional needs. Imagine a dinner where the base meal is a robust vegetable stew. This can be served over a bed of whole-grain rice or buttery mashed potatoes for family members not fasting. Enjoying this stew as is or with a low-carbohydrate base like cauliflower rice might be more in line with your fasting needs. This method allows everyone to feel included and satisfied without requiring you to prepare completely separate meals.

Educating your family about intermittent fasting can also foster understanding and support. It's not uncommon for family members to express concern or curiosity about your new eating pattern. Addressing these thoughts openly can help demystify your choices. Explain the health benefits you're aiming for and how this change could positively impact your well-being. Sharing how fasting fits into your lifestyle might inspire family members, potentially encouraging them to make healthier choices themselves. Moreover, this openness can provide a supportive environment where family members become your cheerleaders, celebrating your dedication and successes.

Inclusive meal planning is another cornerstone of integrating family meals with your fasting schedule. Start with planning meals that naturally align with your eating window. If you typically break your fast around noon, a hearty, late brunch on the weekend can be a wonderful meal for everyone to enjoy together. Dishes like omelets filled with fresh vegetables, cheese, and lean meats offer flexibility; they can be easily customized to suit various taste preferences and are nutritious for both fasting and those who are not.

Flexibility extends to snack times as well. Preparing snacks that fit into your eating window and appeal to children or grandchildren can encourage healthy eating habits across generations. For instance, having cut fruits, nuts, or yogurt available during your eating window provides healthy options that are easy for children to enjoy too. This not only makes your fasting integration smoother but also sets a positive example for younger family members about healthy eating.

The ability to add or subtract components to accommodate everyone's needs without additional hassle is a practical approach to meal planning. For example, if you're preparing a protein like chicken, cook it simply with minimal seasoning. Then, offer a variety of sauces or sides that family members can choose from. Those who are not fasting might opt for a creamy sauce and pasta, while you might choose a lighter vegetable stir-fry or a salad as an accompaniment. This method ensures that the core meal remains the same, but the accompaniments can be tailored to meet individual dietary needs and preferences.

By embracing these strategies—balancing nutritional needs, educating family members, planning inclusive meals, and maintaining flexibility in meal components—you create not just meals but memories that support and enhance your fasting journey while also catering to the well-being of your loved ones. This integration fosters a supportive atmosphere at the dining table, where everyone feels valued and nourished.

As we wrap up this chapter on smart nutrition and meal planning, we've explored how integrating intermittent fasting into your lifestyle doesn't have to be a solo journey. It's very much about community—about sharing meals that bring us together, nourishing our bodies, and celebrating our health.

MAKE A DIFFERENCE WITH YOUR REVIEW

UNLOCK THE POWER OF GENEROSITY

To give and not expect return, that is what lies at the heart of love.

— OSCAR WILDE

People who give without expectation live longer, happier lives and make more money. So if we've got a shot at that during our time together, darn it, I'm gonna try.

To make that happen, I have a question for you...

Would you help someone you've never met, even if you never got credit for it?

Who is this person you ask? They are like you. Or, at least, like you used to be. Less experienced, wanting to make a difference, and needing help, but not sure where to look.

Our mission is to make intermittent fasting accessible to everyone. Everything I do stems from that mission. And, the only way for me to accomplish that mission is by reaching…well…everyone.

This is where you come in. Most people do, in fact, judge a book by its cover (and its reviews). So here's my ask on behalf of a struggling woman over 50 you've never met:

Please help that woman by leaving this book a review.

Your gift costs no money and less than 60 seconds to make real, but can change a fellow reader's life forever. Your review could help…

...one more woman find her way to better health.

...one more reader gain confidence in her journey.

...one more person experience the benefits of intermittent fasting.

To get that 'feel good' feeling and help this person for real, all you have to do is...and it takes less than 60 seconds...

leave a review.

Simply scan the QR code below to leave your review:

For the US	For the UK
SCAN ME	SCAN ME

If you feel good about helping a faceless reader, you are my kind of person. Welcome to the club. You're one of us.

I'm that much more excited to help you achieve your health goals faster and easier than you can possibly imagine. You'll love the tips and strategies I'm about to share in the coming chapters.

Thank you from the bottom of my heart. Now, back to our regularly scheduled programming.

- Your biggest fan, Jennifer Lindsey

PS - Fun fact: If you provide something of value to another person, it makes you more valuable to them. If you'd like goodwill straight from another reader - and you believe this book will help them - send this book their way.

INTERMITTENT FASTING FRIENDLY RECIPES

Whether you're new to intermittent fasting or a seasoned practitioner, the right recipes can significantly improve your experience and results. This chapter is dedicated to providing you with a variety of delicious and nutritious recipes that are perfect for intermittent fasting.

From healthy snacks to satisfying breakfasts, lunches, and dinners, each recipe is crafted to support your fasting routine while keeping your nutritional needs in balance. You'll find options that fit within different calorie ranges, ensuring that you can enjoy flavorful meals whether you're on a fasting day or a regular eating day. Our recipes emphasize high fiber and protein content, essential for maintaining energy levels, supporting muscle repair, and keeping you full longer.

We've also included ketogenic and Mediterranean-friendly options for various dietary preferences. Lean proteins, fish, and plant-based options are highlighted to provide a wide range of choices for every palate. Additionally, you'll discover smoothies, stir-fries, and dishes featuring berries, nuts, and seeds, offering a mix of textures and flavors to keep your meals interesting and enjoyable.

5.1 HEALTHY SNACK OPTIONS

Choosing the right snacks is crucial, and there are plenty of healthy options that are easy to prepare and perfect for consumption within your eating window. Here are a few quick recipes:

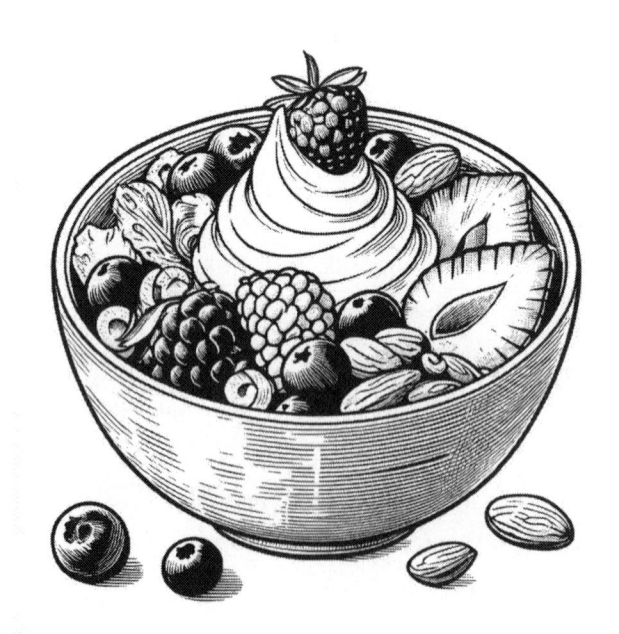

Veggie Sticks with Hummus

Ingredients:

- 1 carrot, sliced into sticks
- 2 celery stalks, sliced into sticks
- 1 bell pepper, sliced into sticks
- 1/2 cup hummus

Instructions:

1. Wash and peel the carrot. Slice it into sticks.
2. Wash the celery stalks and slice them into sticks.
3. Wash the bell pepper, remove the seeds, and slice it into sticks.
4. Arrange the veggie sticks on a plate.
5. Serve with a small bowl of hummus for dipping.

Nutrition: Rich in fiber and protein.

Mixed Nuts and Dried Fruit

Ingredients:

- 1/4 cup mixed nuts (almonds, walnuts, cashews)
- 1/4 cup dried cranberries or apricots

Instructions:

1. Combine the mixed nuts and dried fruit in a small bowl.
2. Mix well to distribute the nuts and fruit evenly.
3. Serve as a satisfying snack with a crunch and a hint of sweetness.

Nutrition: Packed with proteins, fats, and fiber.

Avocado Toast

Ingredients:

- 1 slice of whole-grain bread
- 1/2 avocado, mashed
- A sprinkle of sea salt
- A dash of lime juice

Instructions:

1. Toast the slice of whole-grain bread to your desired level of crispiness.
2. While the bread is toasting, mash the avocado in a small bowl.
3. Spread the mashed avocado evenly over the toasted bread.
4. Sprinkle a pinch of sea salt over the avocado.
5. Add a dash of lime juice for extra flavor.
6. Serve immediately.

Nutrition: Rich in healthy fats and fiber.

Greek Yogurt with Berries and Nuts

Ingredients:

- 1 cup plain Greek yogurt
- 1/2 cup mixed berries (blueberries, raspberries, strawberries)
- 1 tablespoon chopped almonds or walnuts

Instructions:

1. Place the Greek yogurt in a bowl.
2. Top with mixed berries and chopped nuts.
3. Serve immediately.

Swap: Use coconut yogurt as a plant-based option.

Nutrition: High in protein and fiber.

Celery Sticks with Almond Butter

Ingredients:

- 4 celery sticks
- 2 tablespoons almond butter

Instructions:

1. Wash the celery sticks and cut them into halves.
2. Spread almond butter evenly on each celery stick.
3. Serve immediately.

Swap: Use sunflower seed butter for a nut-free option.

Nutrition: High in fiber and healthy fats.

* * *

5.2 BREAKFASTS

Breakfast is often considered the most important meal of the day, providing the necessary energy and nutrients to kickstart your metabolism and maintain focus throughout the morning. Whether you prefer a hearty meal like an omelet or a lighter option like a smoothie, incorporating a balance of protein, fiber, and healthy fats can set a positive tone for the rest of your day.

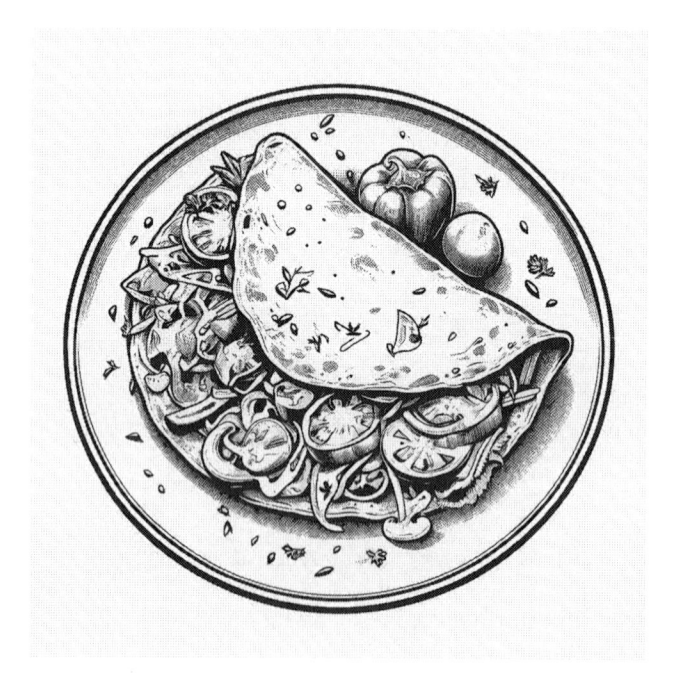

Veggie and Cheese Omelet

Ingredients:

- 2 eggs
- 1/4 cup bell pepper, diced
- 1/4 cup mushrooms, sliced
- 1/4 cup cherry tomatoes, halved
- 1/4 cup shredded cheddar cheese
- 1 tablespoon olive oil
- Salt and pepper to taste

Instructions:

1. Dice, the bell pepper, slice the mushrooms, and halve the cherry tomatoes.
2. Heat the olive oil in a non-stick skillet over medium heat. Add the bell pepper, mushrooms, and cherry tomatoes. Sauté for 3-5 minutes until the vegetables are tender.
3. In a bowl, whisk the eggs with a pinch of salt and pepper.
4. Pour the eggs over the sautéed vegetables in the skillet. Cook until the edges start to set, about 2-3 minutes.
5. Sprinkle the shredded cheddar cheese over the eggs.
6. Fold the omelet in half and cook for another 1-2 minutes until the cheese is melted and the eggs are fully set. Serve immediately.

Swap: Use tofu scramble for a plant-based option.

Nutrition: High in protein and healthy fats, providing a nutritious and satisfying start to your day.

Chia Seed Pudding with Berries

Ingredients:

- 3 tablespoons chia seeds
- 1 cup almond milk
- 1/2 cup mixed berries
- 1 tablespoon honey (optional)

Instructions:

1. In a bowl, mix chia seeds with almond milk.
2. Stir well and refrigerate for at least 4 hours or overnight.
3. Top with mixed berries and honey before serving.

Swap: Use coconut milk for a different flavor.

Nutrition: High in fiber and antioxidants.

Salmon and Avocado Breakfast Bowl

Ingredients:

- 3 oz smoked salmon
- 1/2 avocado, sliced
- 1 cup mixed greens
- 1 tablespoon olive oil
- Lemon juice, salt, and pepper to taste

Instructions:

1. Arrange mixed greens in a bowl.
2. Top with smoked salmon and sliced avocado.

3. Drizzle with olive oil and lemon juice.
4. Season with salt and pepper.
5. Serve immediately.

Nutrition: High in omega-3 fatty acids and protein.

Berry Protein Breakfast Smoothie

Ingredients:

- 1/2 cup mixed berries (strawberries, blueberries, raspberries)
- 1 banana
- 1 cup unsweetened almond milk
- 1/2 cup Greek yogurt
- 1 scoop vanilla protein powder
- 1 tablespoon chia seeds
- 1 handful of spinach (optional for extra nutrients)
- Ice cubes (optional for a thicker smoothie)

Instructions:

1. Wash the mixed berries and spinach (if using). Peel the banana.
2. Combine the mixed berries, banana, almond milk, Greek yogurt, protein powder, chia seeds, and spinach in a blender.
3. Add a few ice cubes if you prefer a thicker smoothie.
4. Blend all ingredients until smooth and creamy.
5. Pour the smoothie into a glass and serve immediately.

Swap: Use green tea instead of Greek yogurt for a lighter option, and consider adding flaxseeds.

Nutrition: High in protein, fiber, and antioxidants, this smoothie provides a balanced and nutritious start to your day, keeping you full and energized.

5.3 LUNCH

Lunch is a crucial meal that helps sustain energy levels and concentration for the rest of the day. Opt for a balanced lunch with lean proteins, whole grains, and plenty of vegetables to keep you satisfied and focused and avoid the afternoon slump.

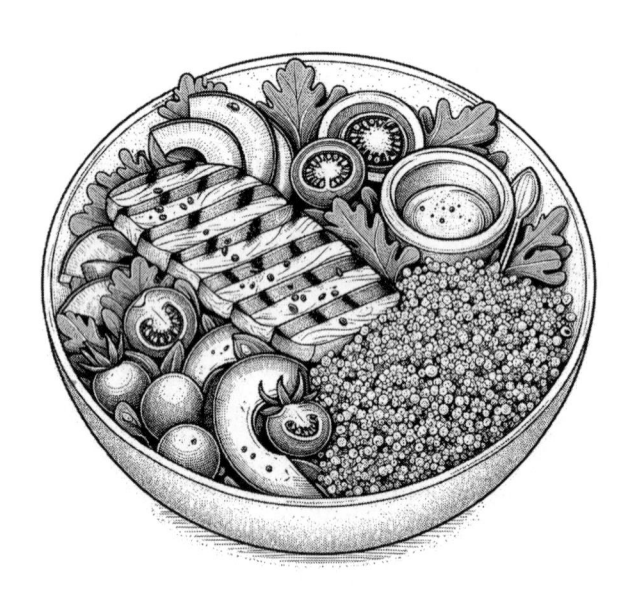

Quinoa Salad with Grilled Chicken

Ingredients:

- 1 cup cooked quinoa
- 4 oz grilled chicken breast, sliced
- 1 cup cherry tomatoes, halved
- 1/2 cucumber, diced
- 1/4 cup crumbled feta cheese
- 2 tablespoons olive oil
- Lemon juice, salt, and pepper to taste

Instructions:

1. Combine quinoa, cherry tomatoes, cucumber, and feta cheese in a large bowl.
2. Add sliced grilled chicken on top.
3. Drizzle with olive oil and lemon juice.
4. Season with salt and pepper.
5. Serve immediately.

Swap: Use tofu or tempeh for a plant-based option.

Nutrition: High in protein and fiber.

Mediterranean Chickpea Salad

Ingredients:

- 1 can chickpeas, drained and rinsed
- 1 cup cherry tomatoes, halved
- 1/2 red onion, finely chopped
- 1/4 cup chopped parsley

- 1/4 cup crumbled feta cheese
- 2 tablespoons olive oil
- Lemon juice, salt, and pepper to taste

Instructions:

1. Combine chickpeas, cherry tomatoes, red onion, and parsley in a large bowl.
2. Add crumbled feta cheese.
3. Drizzle with olive oil and lemon juice.
4. Season with salt and pepper.
5. Serve immediately.

Nutrition: High in fiber and plant-based protein.

Turkey and Avocado Lettuce Wraps

Ingredients:

- 4 large lettuce leaves
- 4 oz sliced turkey breast
- 1/2 avocado, sliced
- 1/2 bell pepper, sliced
- 1 tablespoon hummus

Instructions:

1. Spread hummus on each lettuce leaf.
2. Top with sliced turkey, avocado, and bell pepper.
3. Roll up the lettuce leaves and secure them with toothpicks if necessary.
4. Serve immediately.

Swap: Use tempeh for a plant-based option, or swap for grilled chicken.

Nutrition: High in lean protein and healthy fats.

5.4 DINNER

Dinner is an opportunity to wind down and enjoy a nutritious meal that supports recovery and relaxation after a busy day. Focus on lean proteins, healthy fats, and vegetables to promote restful sleep and provide essential nutrients for overnight recovery.

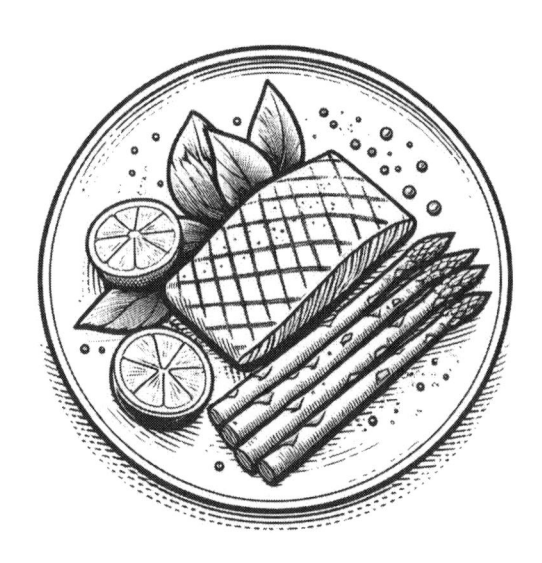

Grilled Salmon with Asparagus

Ingredients:

- 6 oz salmon fillet
- 1 bunch asparagus, trimmed
- 2 tablespoons olive oil
- Lemon slices, salt, and pepper to taste

Instructions:

1. Preheat the grill to medium-high heat.
2. Brush salmon and asparagus with olive oil.
3. Season with salt and pepper.
4. Grill salmon for 5-7 minutes per side until cooked through.
5. Grill asparagus for 3-4 minutes until tender.
6. Serve with lemon slices.

Swap: Use tofu for a plant-based option.

Nutrition: High in omega-3 fatty acids and protein.

Chicken and Vegetable Stir-Fry

Ingredients:

- 4 oz chicken breast, sliced
- 1 cup broccoli florets
- 1 bell pepper, sliced
- 1/2 cup snap peas
- 2 tablespoons soy sauce
- 1 tablespoon olive oil

Instructions:

1. Heat olive oil in a large skillet over medium-high heat.
2. Add sliced chicken and cook until browned.
3. Add broccoli, bell pepper, and snap peas.
4. Stir-fry for 5-7 minutes until vegetables are tender.
5. Add soy sauce and stir to coat.
6. Serve immediately.

Swap: Use tempeh or tofu for a plant-based option.

Nutrition: High in protein and fiber.

Eggplant Parmesan

Ingredients:

- 1 large eggplant, sliced
- 1 cup marinara sauce
- 1 cup shredded mozzarella cheese
- 1/4 cup grated Parmesan cheese
- 2 tablespoons olive oil

Instructions:

1. Preheat oven to 375°F (190°C).
2. Brush eggplant slices with olive oil and place on a baking sheet.
3. Bake for 20 minutes until tender.
4. Layer eggplant slices, marinara sauce, and cheese in a baking dish.
5. Repeat layers and finish with cheese on top.
6. Bake for 20-25 minutes until bubbly and golden.

7. Serve immediately.

Swap: Use vegan cheese for a plant-based option.

Nutrition: High in fiber and plant-based protein.

5.5 MEALS THAT ARE ONLY 500 TO 800 CALORIES

Meals that are only 500 to 800 calories can be both satisfying and nutritious, providing ample energy while helping to manage calorie intake. These meals often include lean proteins, fiber-rich vegetables, and healthy fats, making them ideal for those looking to maintain or achieve a healthy weight without feeling deprived.

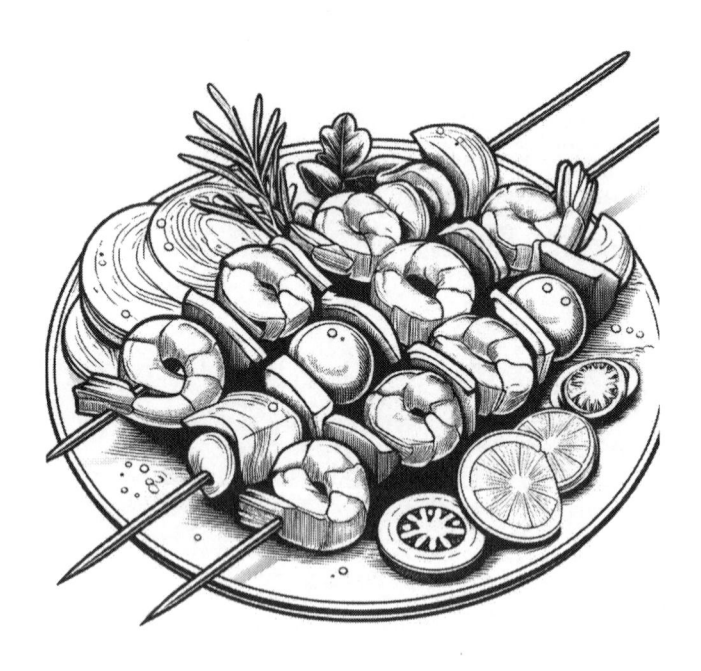

Grilled Shrimp and Veggie Skewers

Ingredients:

- 6 oz shrimp
- 1 bell pepper, cubed
- 1 zucchini, sliced
- 1 tablespoon olive oil
- Lemon juice, salt, and pepper to taste

Instructions:

1. Preheat the grill to medium-high heat.
2. Thread shrimp and vegetables onto skewers.
3. Brush olive oil and season with lemon juice, salt, and pepper.
4. Grill for 5-7 minutes until shrimp are opaque and vegetables are tender.
5. Serve immediately.

Nutrition: High in lean protein and low in calories.

Kale and White Bean Soup

Ingredients:

- 1 can white beans, drained and rinsed
- 2 cups kale, chopped
- 1 carrot, diced
- 1 celery stalk, diced
- 1 tablespoon olive oil
- 4 cups vegetable broth

Instructions:

1. Heat olive oil in a large pot over medium heat.
2. Add diced carrot and celery, and sauté for 5 minutes until softened.
3. Add the white beans and vegetable broth and bring to a boil.
4. Reduce heat, add kale, and simmer for 10 minutes.
5. Season with salt and pepper to taste.
6. Serve hot.

Nutrition: High in fiber and plant-based protein.

Stuffed Bell Peppers

Ingredients:

- 2 bell peppers, halved and seeded
- 1 cup cooked quinoa
- 1/2 cup black beans
- 1/4 cup shredded cheddar cheese
- 1 tablespoon olive oil

Instructions:

1. Preheat oven to 375°F (190°C).
2. Mix cooked quinoa, black beans, and olive oil in a bowl.
3. Stuff the bell pepper halves with the mixture.
4. Top with shredded cheddar cheese.
5. Place stuffed peppers in a baking dish and bake for 25-30 minutes.
6. Serve hot.

Swap: Use lentils instead of black beans for variety.

Nutrition: High in fiber and protein.

Chicken Caesar Salad

Ingredients:

- 4 oz grilled chicken breast
- 2 cups romaine lettuce, chopped
- 1/4 cup grated Parmesan cheese
- 2 tablespoons Caesar dressing
- 1 tablespoon olive oil

Instructions:

1. Chop the romaine lettuce and place it in a bowl.
2. Top with grilled chicken breast slices.
3. Add grated Parmesan cheese and Caesar dressing.
4. Toss the salad to combine.
5. Serve immediately.

Swap: Use tofu for a plant-based option.

Nutrition: High in protein and healthy fats.

Zucchini Noodles with Pesto and Cherry Tomatoes

Ingredients:

- 2 large zucchinis, spiralized
- 1/2 cup cherry tomatoes, halved
- 1/4 cup pesto sauce
- 1 tablespoon olive oil

Instructions:

1. Heat olive oil in a skillet over medium heat.
2. Add zucchini noodles and sauté for 3-4 minutes.
3. Add cherry tomatoes and cook for another 2 minutes.
4. Remove from heat and toss with pesto sauce.
5. Serve immediately.

Swap: Use spaghetti squash for a different texture.

Nutrition: High in fiber and healthy fats.

Baked Cod with Lemon and Herbs

Ingredients:

- 6 oz cod fillet
- 1 lemon, sliced
- 1 tablespoon olive oil
- Fresh herbs (parsley, thyme), salt, and pepper to taste

Instructions:

1. Preheat oven to 400°F (200°C).
2. Place the cod fillet on a baking sheet lined with parchment paper.
3. Drizzle with olive oil and season with salt, pepper, and fresh herbs.
4. Top with lemon slices.
5. Bake for 15-20 minutes until the fish is flaky.
6. Serve hot.

Swap: Use any white fish for variety.

INTERMITTENT FASTING FRIENDLY RECIPES | 99

Nutrition: High in lean protein and omega-3s.

5.6 DAILY MEAL PLAN: 500 TO 600 CALORIES

Here is a completed daily meal plan for a specified calorie range, designed to align with intermittent fasting. It gives an example of the possibilities and ensures high fiber and protein content.

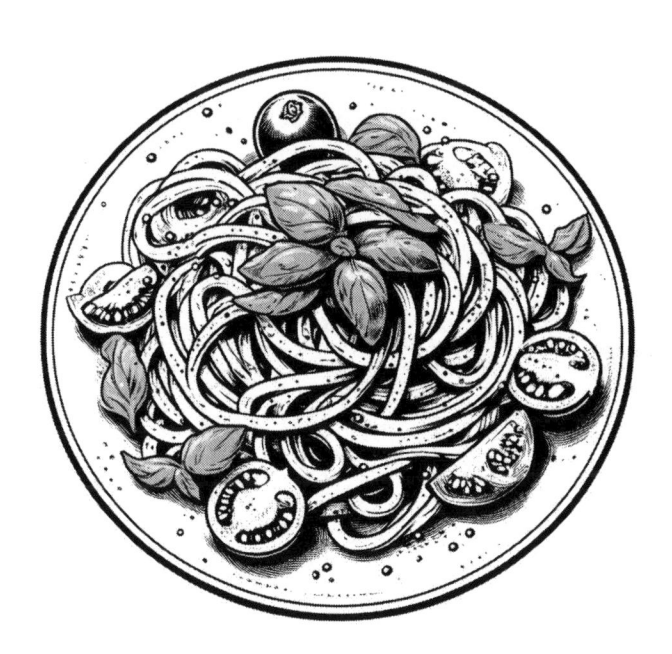

Breakfast: Chia Seed Pudding with Berries

- 3 tablespoons chia seeds (150 calories)
- 1 cup unsweetened almond milk (30 calories)
- 1/2 cup mixed berries (35 calories)

Instructions: Mix chia seeds and almond milk, refrigerate overnight, top with berries before serving.

Total Calories: 215

Lunch: Kale and White Bean Soup

- 1/2 can white beans, drained and rinsed (100 calories)
- 1 cup kale, chopped (33 calories)
- 1/2 carrot, diced (15 calories)
- 1/2 celery stalk, diced (5 calories)
- 1 teaspoon olive oil (40 calories)
- 2 cups vegetable broth (20 calories)

Instructions: Sauté carrot and celery in olive oil, add beans and broth, bring to a boil, add kale, and simmer.

Total Calories: 213

Snack: Celery Sticks with Almond Butter

- 4 celery sticks (10 calories)
- 1 tablespoon almond butter (98 calories)

Instructions: Spread almond butter on celery sticks.

Total Calories: 108

Dinner: Zucchini Noodles with Pesto and Cherry Tomatoes

- 1 large zucchini, spiralized (33 calories)
- 1/4 cup cherry tomatoes, halved (8 calories)
- 2 tablespoons pesto sauce (120 calories)

Instructions: Sauté zucchini noodles in a non-stick pan, add cherry tomatoes, and stir in pesto sauce.

Total Calories: 161

Total Daily Calories: 597

5.7 DAILY MEAL PLAN: 600 TO 800 CALORIES

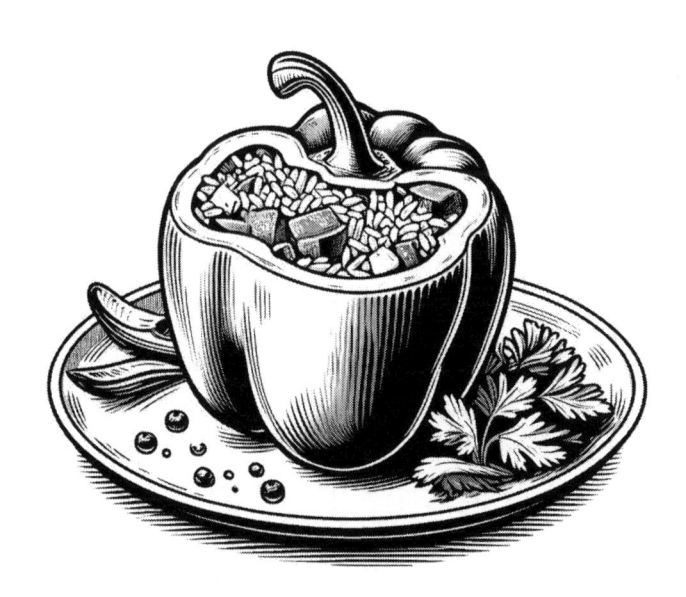

Breakfast: Spinach and Feta Omelet

- 2 eggs (140 calories)
- 1 cup fresh spinach (7 calories)
- 1/4 cup crumbled feta cheese (100 calories)
- 1 teaspoon olive oil (40 calories)

Instructions: Sauté spinach in olive oil, add whisked eggs, cook, and top with feta.

Total Calories: 287

Lunch: Stuffed Bell Peppers

- 1 bell pepper, halved and seeded (25 calories)
- 1/2 cup cooked quinoa (111 calories)
- 1/4 cup black beans (57 calories)
- 2 tablespoons shredded cheddar cheese (55 calories)
- 1 teaspoon olive oil (40 calories)

Instructions: Mix quinoa, beans, and olive oil, stuff peppers, top with cheese, and bake.

Total Calories: 288

Snack: Greek Yogurt with Berries and Nuts

- 1/2 cup plain Greek yogurt (50 calories)
- 1/4 cup mixed berries (17 calories)
- 1 tablespoon chopped almonds or walnuts (50 calories)

Instructions: Mix yogurt, berries, and nuts.

Total Calories: 117

INTERMITTENT FASTING FRIENDLY RECIPES | 103

Dinner: Grilled Shrimp and Veggie Skewers

- 4 oz shrimp (112 calories)
- 1 bell pepper, cubed (25 calories)
- 1 zucchini, sliced (33 calories)
- 1 teaspoon olive oil (40 calories)

Instructions: Thread shrimp and vegetables onto skewers, brush with olive oil, and grill.

Total Calories: 210

Total Daily Calories: 702

5.8 DAILY MEAL PLAN: 800 TO 1000 CALORIES

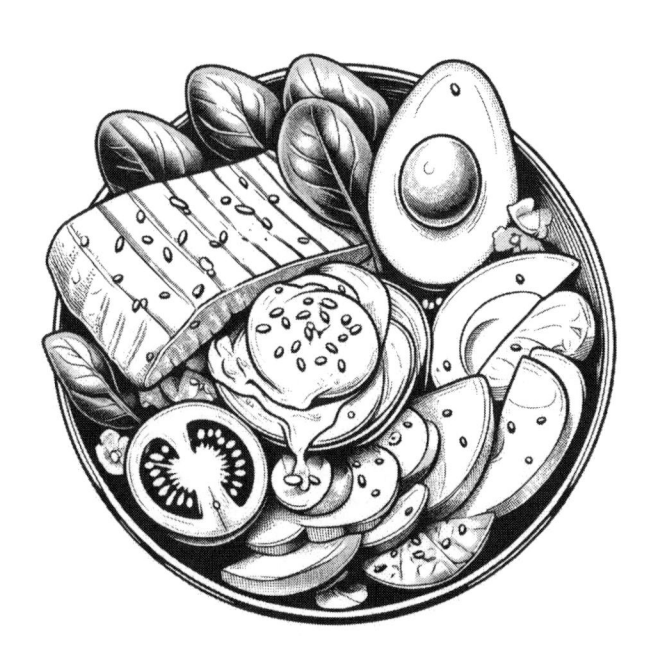

Breakfast: Salmon and Avocado Breakfast Bowl

- 3 oz smoked salmon (133 calories)
- 1/2 avocado, sliced (120 calories)
- 1 cup mixed greens (10 calories)
- 1 teaspoon olive oil (40 calories)
- Lemon juice, salt, and pepper to taste

Instructions: Arrange greens, top with salmon and avocado, drizzle with olive oil and lemon juice.

Total Calories: 303

Lunch: Chicken Caesar Salad

- 4 oz grilled chicken breast (165 calories)
- 2 cups romaine lettuce, chopped (16 calories)
- 1/4 cup grated Parmesan cheese (108 calories)
- 1 tablespoon Caesar dressing (80 calories)

Instructions: Toss lettuce, chicken, Parmesan, and dressing.

Total Calories: 369

Snack: Smoothie with Berries and Spinach

- 1/2 cup mixed berries (35 calories)
- 1 cup spinach (7 calories)
- 1/2 cup unsweetened almond milk (15 calories)
- 1 scoop protein powder (100 calories)

Instructions: Blend all ingredients until smooth.

Total Calories: 157

Dinner: Beef and Broccoli Stir-Fry

- 4 oz beef sirloin, sliced (230 calories)
- 1 cup broccoli florets (55 calories)
- 1 bell pepper, sliced (25 calories)
- 2 tablespoons soy sauce (20 calories)
- 1 tablespoon sesame oil (120 calories)

Instructions: Stir-fry beef in sesame oil, add broccoli and pepper and stir in soy sauce.

Total Calories: 450

Total Daily Calories: 927

The recipes and meal plans offer various delicious and nutritious options that align perfectly with intermittent fasting principles, and ketogenic and Mediterranean diets. By carefully selecting ingredients rich in protein, fiber, and healthy fats, these meals ensure you receive essential nutrients even when reducing portion sizes. This approach supports overall health and aids in weight management and maintaining energy levels throughout the day.

Even with a caloric intake of up to 1000 calories, these well-balanced meals are designed to keep you full and satisfied. The strategic combination of lean proteins, fiber-dense vegetables, and healthy fats helps to prolong satiety, preventing hunger pangs and energy dips. Focusing on nutrient-dense foods allows you to enjoy flavorful meals that meet your dietary needs, support your fasting routine, and promote a sustainable, healthy lifestyle. Next, we focus on overcoming challenges and setbacks, aiming to arm you with strategies to maintain your fasting schedule with confidence and ease, regardless of the hurdles that come your way.

OVERCOMING CHALLENGES AND SETBACKS

Imagine you're on a serene hiking trail, the path stretching before you, lined with the promise of lush vistas and stimulating experiences. As with any adventure, there are occasional obstacles—a fallen log across the path, a sudden steep incline, or a misleading fork in the road. The journey of intermittent fasting, much like hiking, isn't without its challenges. However, with the right strategies and mindset, these hurdles can be navigated successfully, leading you to your desired health and wellness destination.

6.1 HANDLING HUNGER PANGS: TIPS AND TRICKS

Understanding Hunger Signals

Understanding your body's signals is crucial in distinguishing between true hunger and mere habitual eating cues or emotional cravings. Physiologically, hunger is your body's natural way of telling you it needs fuel, typically signaled by a growling stomach, a slight headache, or even feelings of weakness. On the other hand, psychological hunger is driven by factors such as stress, boredom, or external cues like the sight or smell of food, which can lead to mindless eating. Recognizing these signs and learning to respond appropriately is a crucial step in managing your fasting effectively.

Strategies to Mitigate Hunger

When accurate hunger strikes, especially during the early days of adapting to your fasting schedule, knowing how to mitigate these feelings can make a significant difference. One practical approach is to consume high-volume, low-calorie foods during your eating window. Foods like leafy greens, cucumbers, and broth-based soups can fill you up without consuming too many calories. Incorporating fiber-rich foods such as legumes and whole grains can also prolong feelings of fullness.

Another useful strategy is the use of natural appetite suppressants. A cup of green tea or black coffee, for instance, can provide a comforting ritual, and temporarily reduce your appetite, thanks to its caffeine content and other bioactive compounds. Furthermore, engaging in distraction techniques can be incredibly effective. When hunger pangs strike, try diverting your attention with a walk, a book, or a hobby that keeps your hands and mind busy, shifting your focus away from food.

Timing Nutrient Intake

Strategically planning your nutrient intake during your eating window can also significantly extend satiety and make your fasting periods more manageable. Prioritizing protein intake can be particularly effective, as proteins are known to increase levels of satiety-inducing hormones. Eating a protein-rich meal as your last meal before starting a fast, for example, can help ensure that your hunger pangs are kept at bay for longer during the fasting period.

Psychological Coping Mechanisms

Adopting psychological strategies is critical to managing the mental challenge of hunger during fasting. Mindful eating practices can transform your relationship with food. This means paying full attention to the eating process, savoring each bite, and acknowledging the flavors, textures, and sensations involved, which can help in recognizing satiety cues more effectively.

Cognitive reframing is another powerful tool. This involves changing your perspective on hunger. Instead of viewing hunger pangs as unbearable or a signal of deprivation, try to see them as positive signs that your body is transitioning into a fat-burning state, a step toward achieving your health goals. This shift in mindset can reduce the discomfort associated with hunger and can make your fasting journey more pleasant.

Interactive Element: Journaling Prompt

Maintain a hunger diary to enhance your understanding and management of hunger. Note the times when you feel hungry, the intensity of your hunger, what you eat, and how you feel afterward. Over time, this can help you identify patterns in your hunger signals and more effectively strategize your eating and fasting periods. This self-awareness tool not only aids in personalizing your fasting approach but also empowers you to take control of your eating behaviors, aligning them more closely with your body's true needs.

In navigating the challenges of intermittent fasting, remember that each step, whether forward or slightly backward, is part of a more significant journey toward a healthier you. By understanding and managing hunger effectively, employing strategic eating practices, and adopting a positive psychological approach, you can turn the challenges of intermittent fasting into stepping stones for success. As you continue to adapt and learn, overcoming each challenge adds confidence and empowerment, enhancing your ability to maintain this healthful practice long-term.

6.2 SOCIAL EATING AND INTERMITTENT FASTING: HOW TO BALANCE BOTH

Navigating social events while maintaining your intermittent fasting schedule can sometimes feel like trying to dance the waltz to a rock song—there's a bit of a mismatch in rhythm. However, with some planning and communication, you can gracefully manage your social engagements without sidestepping your health goals. Let's explore some strategies to help you maintain your fasting routine while enjoying the company of friends and family over meals.

Planning Ahead for Social Events

Anticipating social occasions and planning accordingly can make a significant difference. If you know a birthday party or family gathering is coming up, consider adjusting your fasting schedule in advance. For instance, if your usual eating window closes at 6 PM but the event is at 7 PM, you might shift your window to close at 8 PM that day. This minor adjustment allows you to engage in the event thoroughly and enjoy a meal with loved ones without breaking your fasting protocol. It's all about flexibility within structure; intermittent fasting should fit into your life, not dictate it rigidly. Pre-planning these adjustments not only keeps you on track but also reduces stress, letting you focus on enjoying the moment.

Communication Tips

Clear communication is vital when it comes to dietary preferences, especially in a social setting. There's a fine line between sharing your choices and feeling as though you're defending them. If dietary topics come up, keep your explanations simple and positive. You might say, "I've found eating this way really works for me right now," which keeps the conversation light and centered on your personal choice without implying judgment of others' eating habits. This approach can help in maintaining social harmony and making others comfortable with your dietary preferences. It also opens up a space where curiosity leads to supportive dialogues rather than critical ones.

Choosing Suitable Dining Options

Whether you're dining out or eating at a friend's place, selecting suitable menu items that align with your nutritional needs and fasting schedule can help you stay on track. Most restaurants offer a variety of dishes that can cater to different dietary preferences. Look for meals that are rich in proteins and vegetables, which can help you feel full longer and provide essential nutrients without excessive calories. If the menu isn't flexible, consider eating a small, nutritionally balanced snack before you go. This way, you can still enjoy small portions of what's offered without becoming too hungry or feeling like you're missing out.

Handling Peer Pressure

Sometimes, well-meaning friends or family may encourage you to eat outside your fasting window or choose foods that don't align with your goals. This is where having a few polite but firm responses can be handy. You might say, "I appreciate your concern, but I feel great with my current eating schedule," or "Thank you for offering, but I'm really enjoying the way I'm eating right now." These responses acknowledge the other person's care or effort while reinforcing your commitment to your health choices. Remember, staying true to your health goals and respecting your body's needs should always take precedence, and most people will respect your preferences when you communicate them confidently and respectfully.

Navigating social settings while maintaining an intermittent fasting schedule doesn't have to be a source of stress. With thoughtful planning, clear communication, and strategic choices, you can enjoy the best of both worlds—nurturing your social relationships and honoring your health commitments. As you continue to integrate these practices, you'll find that managing social eating becomes more straightforward and more natural, allowing you to stay focused on your health goals without sacrificing meaningful moments with friends and family.

6.3 DEALING WITH PLATEAUS: NEXT STEPS WHEN WEIGHT LOSS STALLS

In the pursuit of any significant health goal, there often comes a time when progress seems to stall stubbornly. This plateau, a common experience in weight loss journeys, can feel particularly disheartening. Imagine you're climbing a hill, steadily making your way to the top, when suddenly, the path levels out, and no matter how hard you push, you can't seem to find your way upward. Understanding why these plateaus occur and how to navigate through them can help rekindle your momentum and renew your commitment to your health goals.

Identifying a Plateau

Recognizing when you've hit a plateau is the first step in overcoming it. Typically, a weight loss plateau is defined as a period where there's no significant change in body weight for two or more weeks despite sticking to your diet and exercise routine. But plateaus can manifest in other aspects of health improvement, too, such as stalls in muscle gain or no further improvements in blood sugar levels. Common reasons for plateaus include metabolic adaptations as your body becomes more efficient at using energy and decreased caloric needs as your body weight decreases. Understanding that plateaus are a normal part of the process can provide some comfort and reassurance that you're not alone in this experience.

Strategic Adjustments in Fasting

Adjusting your intermittent fasting strategy is one effective way to break through a weight loss plateau. If you've been following the same fasting schedule for a while, your body might have adapted to it. Shifting your fasting windows, perhaps by extending them or changing your eating periods, can help restart weight loss. For instance, if you've been comfortable with the 16/8 method, pushing it to 18/6 might provide a new challenge for your metabolism. Alternatively, incorporating a full 24-hour fast once a week could help shake things up. These adjustments can help reignite your body's fat-burning capabilities.

Another strategic approach is to introduce periodic longer fasts, which can help deepen your fasting state and enhance autophagy, the body's way of cleaning out damaged cells. This not only aids in weight management but also contributes to improved overall health. However, these should be approached cautiously and, ideally, under the guidance of a healthcare professional, especially if you have underlying health conditions.

Reassessing Caloric Needs

As you lose weight, your body requires fewer calories to function than it did at your heavier weight. This reduced caloric need might be contributing to your weight loss stall. It's essential to reassess your caloric needs periodically, especially after losing significant weight. Tools like the basal metabolic rate (BMR) calculators can help estimate your daily calorie needs based on your current weight, age, gender, and activity level. Adjusting your calorie intake according to your new metabolic needs can help overcome a plateau by ensuring you are in a caloric deficit, which is conducive to continued weight loss.

Incorporating Resistance Training

Adding resistance training to your routine can be a game-changer in managing a weight loss plateau. Resistance exercises help build muscle mass, which burns more calories than fat even when you're at rest, thus boosting your metabolism. More muscle mass means your body uses energy more efficiently, which can help break through a weight loss stall. Engaging in weight lifting, resistance bands, or body-weight exercises such as push-ups, squats, and lunges can significantly enhance your strength and muscle tone, supporting your weight loss efforts.

Incorporating these strategies into your routine requires patience and persistence, but the rewards can be substantial. Adjusting your fasting schedule, reassessing your caloric needs, and adding resistance training are practical steps you can take to overcome the inevitable plateaus in your health improvement journey. As you implement these changes, remember to monitor your progress and continue adjusting your approach based on what works best for your body. This proactive attitude can help you maintain your motivation and commitment to achieving your health goals, navigating past the plateaus to continue on your path to wellness.

6.4 ADJUSTING YOUR FASTING SCHEDULE AROUND MEDICAL NEEDS

As you weave intermittent fasting into the fabric of your daily life, it's crucial to remember that your health journey may have unique turns, especially if you're managing ongoing medical conditions or prescribed medications. Collaborating closely with healthcare providers is helpful and essential in these circumstances. Think of your doctor as a trusted guide who helps you navigate through a landscape dotted with medical needs, ensuring that your fasting schedule enhances your health without compromising it.

The interplay between fasting periods and medication schedules can be complex when managing medications. Certain medications require food to aid absorption or to mitigate potential side effects. Here's where the invaluable guidance of your healthcare provider comes into play. They can help you adjust the timing of your medications so that they align harmoniously with your eating windows. For instance, if you're used to taking medication in the morning but your eating window doesn't start until noon, your doctor might suggest an alternative medication that can be taken on an empty stomach or adjust the timing to fit within your feeding period.

For those navigating chronic conditions such as diabetes, hypertension, or heart disease, tailoring your fasting approach is particularly critical. Each of these conditions has nuances that may require specific adjustments in your fasting routine. For example, if you have diabetes, monitoring your blood sugar levels becomes paramount. Fasting can influence insulin sensitivity and glucose production, so having a customized fasting plan that considers your blood sugar patterns is crucial. Your healthcare provider can help you determine the safest fasting methods and durations and may even suggest regularly monitoring your glucose levels at home.

Monitoring health markers regularly is another pillar in safely adapting fasting to fit medical needs. Regular check-ups where you can discuss your blood pressure, cholesterol levels, and other relevant health metrics with your doctor are vital. These metrics can provide you and your healthcare provider with insights into how well your body responds to intermittent fasting and whether any adjustments are needed for your specific health circumstances. This ongoing surveillance acts like a feedback loop, offering timely data to help fine-tune your fasting routine to better support your health goals and medical needs.

Navigating intermittent fasting with medical considerations in mind ensures that your fasting approach is proactive and protective. By staying engaged with your healthcare provider, adjusting medication timings as needed, and tailoring fasting practices to accommodate any chronic conditions, you can embrace intermittent fasting as a supportive part of your overall health strategy. This thoughtful customization ensures that your path to wellness is both safe and effective, respecting your body's needs and the medical advice designed to guide you.

6.5 EMOTIONAL EATING VS. SCHEDULED EATING: ESTABLISHING CONTROL

Navigating the complex terrain of emotional eating versus physical hunger is akin to learning to identify the subtle notes in a complex melody. Often, the lines between eating out of emotional need and eating because our bodies genuinely require nourishment can blur, making it difficult to distinguish one from the other. Emotional eating often stems from seeking comfort or suppressing unpleasant emotions with food, which can disrupt your intermittent fasting schedule and undermine your health goals. Recognizing these triggers is the first step in cultivating a healthier relationship with food.

Emotional hunger can be sneaky; it suddenly demands instant satisfaction with specific cravings, like something sweet or salty, which physical hunger does not. It's also not located in the stomach but rather in your head, often accompanied by an emotional void. Unlike physical hunger, which increases gradually and can be satisfied with any food, emotional hunger urges you to eat more even when you are full, leading to feelings of guilt or shame afterward. Learning to recognize these signs is crucial. It helps you understand whether you're eating to satisfy an emotional need or to nourish your body.

One effective strategy to manage emotional eating involves integrating stress management techniques into your daily routine. Activities such as yoga, meditation, or even simple breathing exercises can significantly alleviate the stress that often triggers emotional eating. These practices help reduce stress and enhance your overall well-being, making you less likely to turn to food for emotional comfort. Moreover, establishing a supportive network of friends or family members who understand and support your goals can provide the emotional sustenance that you might otherwise seek from food. Sharing your experiences, challenges, and successes with them can provide encouragement and alternative perspectives, helping you manage emotional triggers more effectively.

Setting a structured eating schedule within your intermittent fasting framework is pivotal in combating emotional eating. Eating at regular intervals can stabilize blood sugar levels, which helps reduce mood swings and improves your overall emotional and physical response to hunger. This doesn't mean you can't be flexible; instead, it's about creating a loose structure that helps prevent random snacking or emotional eating binges. For instance, if your eating window is from 12 pm to 8 pm, you might plan to have a hearty meal right at noon, a balanced snack at 3 pm, and then dinner at 7 pm. This schedule not only covers your nutritional bases but also provides little room for unplanned eating, which is often emotional.

For those who find that emotional eating is a recurrent, disruptive force, it may be beneficial to seek professional help. Consulting with a psychologist or counselor skilled in dealing with eating disorders or emotional eating issues can be incredibly beneficial. These professionals can offer strategies tailored to your personal experiences, helping you delve deeper into the emotional roots of your eating behaviors. Therapy can provide you with tools to cope with emotions in healthier ways, reducing your reliance on food for emotional comfort.

Incorporating these strategies into your life requires patience and persistence, but the benefits extend far beyond your eating habits. You transform your relationship with food by managing emotional eating effectively, setting a structured eating schedule, and seeking professional help when needed. It becomes less about feeding your emotions and more about nourishing your body and soul. This shift not only supports your intermittent fasting efforts but also enhances your overall quality of life, ensuring that food holds its proper place as a source of nourishment and pleasure, not a band-aid for emotional wounds. As you continue to practice these strategies, remember that each day is a new opportunity to reinforce these healthy habits, steadily moving towards a more balanced and fulfilling relationship with food.

6.6 FASTING DURING HOLIDAYS AND SPECIAL OCCASIONS

Navigating holidays and special occasions while maintaining an intermittent fasting schedule can often feel like fitting a square peg into a round hole. The festive seasons are replete with culinary temptations and social gatherings centered around food, making it challenging to stick to your fasting routine. However, with some foresight and flexible strategies, you can enjoy these celebratory times without compromising your health goals.

Pre-emptive Planning

Approaching holidays with a plan can make a significant difference. Before the festive season begins, take a moment to look at your calendar. Identify key dates and events that might pose challenges to your fasting schedule. Once you have a clear view, you can start strategizing. For example, if you know you have a family dinner extending beyond your usual eating window, you might shift your fasting period for that day. Alternatively, if a full day of festivities is planned, you might decide to break your fast earlier or extend it the following day. The key is to prepare these adjustments in advance rather than making spur-of-the-moment decisions, which can lead to unintentionally breaking your fasting goals.

Flexible Fasting Protocols

Flexibility during the holidays is crucial. Introducing more adaptable fasting protocols during these times can help you maintain your overall progress without feeling restricted. One approach is the 5:2 method, where you might typically eat normally for five days and restrict calories on 2 days. During a festive week, you could adjust this to fit your social commitments—perhaps fasting more strictly on quieter days and allowing more flexibility on celebration days. This method helps manage caloric intake over the week and aligns with the ebb and flow of social festivities, allowing you to partake in the joy of the season without guilt.

Mindful Eating During Celebrations

When you do partake in festive meals, embracing mindful eating practices can immensely enhance your experience. This means being fully present at the moment, savoring each bite, and paying attention to flavors and textures. It's about quality, not quantity. Enjoy the unique dishes that are meaningful to you and your family, but do so in moderation. Focusing on portion control can help you enjoy a variety of festive foods without overindulging. For instance, if you love both mashed potatoes and stuffing, you might choose a smaller portion of each rather than a whole serving. By eating slowly and deliberately, you allow yourself the pleasure of tasting all the flavors without the need to overeat.

Returning to Routine

After the holidays, transitioning back to your regular fasting schedule is just as important as planning for the break. This can sometimes be challenging, especially if your routine significantly differs during the holidays. To make this transition smoother, consider setting short-term, achievable goals to regain your fasting rhythm. Start with a gentle approach, perhaps reintroducing shorter fasting periods and gradually increasing them to your usual routine over a few days. This gradual approach helps your body readjust without the shock of a sudden change, making it easier to reestablish your fasting habits.

Navigating fasting during holidays and special occasions requires a balance of planning, flexibility, and mindfulness. By anticipating challenges, adapting your fasting approach to accommodate special days, enjoying festive foods mindfully, and easing back into your routine, you can maintain your health goals without missing out on the joy and traditions that make these times special. As you move forward, these strategies make your fasting journey more adaptable and enjoyable, reflecting the dynamic nature of life's celebrations.

As this chapter closes, remember that the essence of overcoming challenges in intermittent fasting, whether they are hunger pangs, social settings, or holiday feasts, lies in thoughtful preparation, flexible adjustment, and a deep understanding of your body's needs. These strategies are not just about maintaining a fasting schedule; they are about enriching your life with health and vitality, no matter the season. Moving forward, the next chapter will explore sustaining long-term success with intermittent fasting, building on the foundations we've established and looking towards a future where fasting becomes a seamless part of your lifestyle.

PHYSICAL ACTIVITY AND INTERMITTENT FASTING

Imagine you're embarking on a scenic hike; with each step, you're not just moving forward; you're enhancing your strength, endurance, and vitality. This chapter is akin to preparing for that hike, equipping you with the best practices in physical activity that synergize beautifully with your intermittent fasting routine. Just as different trails offer unique challenges and rewards, various forms of exercise complement your fasting lifestyle in distinct ways. Here, we explore how to integrate physical activity into your routine, ensuring it matches your body's needs and fasting schedule, ultimately helping you enjoy a fuller, more energetic life.

7.1 THE BEST TYPES OF EXERCISE TO PAIR WITH INTERMITTENT FASTING

The synergy between intermittent fasting and exercise is akin to a well-orchestrated dance, each step calculated to enhance the other. When you combine exercise with intermittent fasting, they work together to amplify fat loss, improve metabolic health, and increase growth hormone levels, which are crucial for maintaining lean muscle mass and vitality. This interplay is particularly beneficial as you navigate the changes your body undergoes in your fifties and beyond.

Synergistic Effects of Exercise and IF

When you exercise during your fasting period, your body has already begun to lower its insulin levels and tap into fat reserves for energy, a state known as increased lipolysis. Physical activity during this time can accelerate fat burning, as your body is primed to utilize fat for fuel. Moreover, fasting leads to elevated levels of norepinephrine, further enhancing your body's ability to break down fat. This process not only aids in weight loss but also improves your metabolic flexibility, allowing your body to switch more efficiently between using carbs and fats as fuel sources. Additionally, exercise during fasting has been shown to significantly boost human growth hormone levels, which helps preserve muscle mass—a concern for many women over 50, especially during calorie restriction phases.

Recommended Exercise Types

Aerobic exercises, also known as cardio, are fantastic during fasting periods as they are effective and sustainable methods for burning fat. Activities like walking, cycling, and swimming are particularly beneficial because they can be done at a moderate intensity, which is ideal for burning fat without overstressing your body. These types of exercises increase your heart rate and breathing, encouraging the flow of blood and oxygen throughout your body, which not only aids in fat loss but also improves cardiovascular health and increases stamina.

Strength Training Benefits

While the benefits of aerobic exercise are widely promoted, strength training is equally important, especially for women over 50. Resistance training helps build and preserve muscle mass, which naturally declines with age. Maintaining muscle is crucial not only for strength and mobility but also because muscle tissue burns more calories at rest compared to fat tissue, thus helping to prevent the metabolic slowdown associated with aging. Incorporating strength training into your routine can include using light weights, resistance bands, or body-weight exercises such as modified push-ups, chair squats, and gentle lunges. Regular strength training can strengthen bones, manage weight, and reduce the risk of chronic diseases like diabetes and heart disease.

Tailoring Exercise Intensity

Adjusting the intensity and timing of your workouts to align with your fasting schedule is critical to maximizing the benefits while ensuring your body recovers properly. If you're new to combining fasting with exercise, start with lower-intensity workouts to see how your body responds. It's essential to listen to your body and provide it with adequate nutrition during your eating windows to support recovery. For example, scheduling more intense workouts during or just before your eating periods can help ensure that your post-workout meals aid recovery by replenishing glycogen stores and providing protein for muscle repair.

7.2 LOW-IMPACT WORKOUTS FOR SUSTAINABLE HEALTH

As you gracefully navigate the later chapters of your wellness story, low-impact exercises emerge as unsung heroes, perfectly attuned to your body's evolving needs. Embracing such activities can be a game-changer, significantly enhancing your fitness without overtaxing your joints or risking injury. These types of workouts are gentle yet effective, making them ideal for maintaining your fitness as you integrate intermittent fasting into your lifestyle.

Low-impact exercises are designed to minimize the stress on your body, particularly your joints. By reducing the impact of each movement, these exercises lower the risk of injury. They are particularly beneficial if you have existing joint issues or are just starting to incorporate more physical activity into your life. But don't let the term "low-impact" fool you; these exercises pack a powerful punch for enhancing cardiovascular health, improving muscular strength, and boosting endurance. They are particularly advantageous as they allow you to maintain a consistent exercise routine, which is crucial for metabolic health, especially when paired with intermittent fasting. The beauty of low-impact workouts lies in their ability to provide a sustainable way to exercise, ensuring you can continue to move and stay active, celebrating your body's capability without the fear of pain or injury.

Let's explore some practical low-impact workouts that you can easily incorporate into your weekly routine. Pilates, for instance, is a fantastic option focusing on core strength, flexibility, and overall body alignment. Pilates exercises are performed either on a mat or using special equipment like a reformer, which provides resistance. The movements are slow, controlled, and deliberate, emphasizing quality over quantity, which makes Pilates an excellent choice for strengthening your muscles and enhancing your posture without unnecessary strain on your joints.

Another great low-impact activity is aqua aerobics. Performed in a swimming pool, aqua aerobics utilizes the natural resistance of water to strengthen your muscles while buoyancy reduces the strain on your joints. This makes it an excellent workout, particularly if you enjoy being in the water. The water resistance makes the exercises more challenging than they might seem, providing a fantastic cardiovascular workout while being gentle on the body.

Elliptical training is also worth considering. Elliptical machines provide a smooth, flowing motion that mimics walking or running without a high impact on your knees and hips. This equipment allows you to adjust the intensity and incline, letting you customize your workout according to your fitness level and goals. It's an effective way to boost your heart rate and burn calories, all while keeping the stress off your lower body.

Incorporating these workouts into your weekly routine requires a balanced approach. Aim to mix different types of low-impact exercises to keep your routine interesting and cover various aspects of fitness. For instance, you might schedule Pilates classes twice a week for strength and flexibility, aqua aerobics once a week for a fun, cardiovascular challenge, and use the elliptical machine in between for endurance building. It's essential to listen to your body and adjust the frequency, intensity, and type of exercise according to how you feel. This approach helps prevent fatigue and keeps your exercise routine enjoyable and sustainable.

Monitoring Impact on Health

Consider using a fitness tracker or a heart rate monitor to ensure you're exercising within a safe and effective range. These tools can be incredibly helpful in keeping track of your exertion levels, heart rate, and the number of calories burned during each workout. They provide valuable feedback to help you adjust your intensity to stay within a target heart rate zone, optimizing your efforts and ensuring you get the most out of your workouts without overdoing it. Tracking your activity also helps in maintaining consistency, which is critical for building and sustaining fitness, especially when combined with intermittent fasting.

As you integrate these low-impact workouts into your life, they do more than just improve your physical health. They enhance your energy levels, boost your mood, and contribute to a greater sense of well-being, proving that taking care of your body is not just about high-impact, high-intensity activities. It's about finding joy in movements that respect your body's limits and capabilities, allowing you to thrive at any age.

7.3 YOGA AND MINDFULNESS: ENHANCING MENTAL AND PHYSICAL HEALTH

Embracing yoga during your intermittent fasting routine can feel like discovering a secret garden—a tranquil space where each movement and breath brings you closer to a state of harmony and balance. Yoga isn't just about bending and stretching; it's about forging a deep connection between mind and body, enhancing both your physical flexibility and mental clarity. This holistic approach is particularly beneficial when paired with intermittent fasting, as it supports both the physical transformations and the cognitive shifts that come with this lifestyle change.

Yoga offers dual benefits, making it an invaluable part of your health routine. Physically, yoga enhances flexibility, strengthens muscles, and can improve your posture, which, for many women over 50, is crucial for maintaining mobility and reducing the risk of falls and injuries. But the benefits extend beyond the physical. Yoga is a powerful tool for stress reduction and mental clarity. The mindful nature of yoga—focusing on the present moment and the flow of breath—helps to quiet the mind and reduce stress. This mental clarity is crucial when you're adjusting to a new eating pattern, helping you stay committed and mindful of your body's cues. During fasting, when some experience mild stress or irritability, yoga can serve as a soothing balm, helping to keep your emotions balanced and stress levels in check.

Types of Yoga for Different Needs

Yoga comes in various styles, each offering different intensities and focuses, making it accessible for everyone, regardless of fitness level or experience. Hatha yoga is an excellent choice for those new to yoga or looking for a gentle practice. Hatha is often slower-paced and focuses on basic poses and breathing techniques, making it ideal for beginners or those interested in a more meditative practice. This style is particularly beneficial for those fasting, as it does not overly tax the body and aligns well with the energy levels typically experienced during fasting periods.

On days when you feel more energetic and want to challenge yourself, Vinyasa yoga might be the perfect fit. Known for its fluid, movement-intensive practices, Vinyasa links breath with motion in a series of poses that build strength and endurance. This style can be more vigorous, providing a cardiovascular benefit as you move continuously from one pose to another. Vinyasa is particularly effective at boosting metabolism, complementing the metabolic changes induced by intermittent fasting, and enhancing the fat-burning process.

For those who seek to improve balance and core strength, Iyengar yoga, with its emphasis on precision and alignment, might be appealing. This form of yoga uses props like blocks, straps, and bolsters to help achieve and hold poses for longer periods. This not only enhances your physical alignment and posture but also teaches you patience and focus, qualities that are beneficial when adapting to the discipline of intermittent fasting.

Mindfulness Practices

Integrating mindfulness techniques into your yoga practice can enhance the benefits of your exercise and fasting routine. Mindfulness involves staying present and fully engaging in the moment without judgment. This can be practiced through meditation, where you focus on your breath while observing the thoughts and sensations that arise, allowing them to pass without attachment. Another mindfulness practice, controlled breathing or pranayama, involves directing your attention to your breath pattern, which can help manage stress and reduce anxiety. These practices enhance mental clarity, making it easier to cope with the hunger and energy fluctuations that can come with fasting.

Creating a Yoga Routine

Starting a yoga routine might seem daunting, but it doesn't have to be. Begin by exploring different classes in your local area or online to find a style and instructor that resonates with you. Many community centers, gyms, and yoga studios offer classes specifically designed for older adults, which can accommodate different physical limitations and provide a great way to meet others on a similar path. If you prefer practicing at home, numerous online platforms offer a range of yoga classes that can be done in your living room. Creating a serene space at home for your practice can also help make yoga a regular part of your routine. Find a quiet corner, lay down a comfortable yoga mat, perhaps light a candle or some incense, and let this space be your retreat, where you can come to reconnect and recharge.

Incorporating yoga and mindfulness into your lifestyle enhances your physical health by improving flexibility and strength and supports your mental health, reducing stress and improving focus. This holistic approach is especially beneficial when combined with intermittent fasting, helping to manage the physical and emotional challenges that come with adjusting to a new eating pattern. As you continue to explore and integrate these practices into your life, they can become powerful tools in maintaining your overall health and well-being, allowing you to engage more fully in every moment.

7.4 SCHEDULING WORKOUTS: BEST TIMES DURING YOUR FASTING CYCLE

When integrating exercise with intermittent fasting, timing can be just as crucial as the type of workout you choose. It's much like tuning an instrument; finding the right balance can help you play the most harmonious tune. Many of you have probably wondered about the best time to exercise during your fasting cycle and how to align your workouts with your energy levels and meal timings. Let's explore how to strategically schedule your workouts to enhance both fat loss and muscle synthesis, ensuring you maintain high energy levels and efficient recovery.

Optimal Timing for Energy Levels

Understanding your body's natural rhythms and how they interact with your fasting schedule is critical to optimizing your workout timing. Generally, our energy levels tend to peak mid-morning to early afternoon. This window is often ideal for scheduling workouts because your body's metabolism is in full swing, and you're likely to perform better and recover faster. However, every woman's body is unique, especially over the age of 50, as hormonal changes can affect energy levels. It's important to monitor how you feel during different times of the day and adjust your workout schedule accordingly. Some may find that a brisk walk or a light jog in the morning feels invigorating and sets a positive tone for the day, while others might discover that an afternoon session of strength training is more suitable when their body feels more warmed up and responsive.

Fasted vs. Fed State Exercise

The debate between fasted and fed state exercise is ongoing, but both have unique advantages depending on your goals and physical condition. Exercising in a fasted state, typically before your first meal, can help maximize your body's fat-burning capabilities. During fasting, lowered insulin levels and depleted glycogen stores force your body to burn more fat for fuel. This can be particularly effective if you're aiming to lose weight. However, fed-state exercises might be more beneficial if you aim to build or preserve muscle mass. Eating before exercising provides you with the energy necessary for intensive strength training, and it helps stimulate muscle protein synthesis during and after your workout, which is essential for muscle growth and repair.

Adjusting Schedules as Needed

Life is unpredictable, and so is our response to diet and exercise, particularly during different phases of life. As you progress with intermittent fasting, it's vital to remain flexible and adjust your workout times based on your body's feedback. If you notice prolonged fatigue or lack of progress in your fitness goals, it could be a sign that your body is not recovering adequately between fasts and workouts. Consider shifting your exercises to your eating windows when you have more energy and can refuel your body immediately afterward. Additionally, tracking your performance and how you feel after each workout can provide valuable insights, helping you tweak your schedule to better suit your needs.

Example Schedules

To give you a practical framework, here are a couple of sample schedules aligning different types of workouts with various intermittent fasting plans:

1. **16/8 Fasting Plan**: If your eating window is from 12 pm to 8 pm, consider a mid-morning workout around 10 am for a fasted cardio session, which can enhance fat burning. Alternatively, schedule a strength training session at 6 pm, allowing you to consume a protein-rich post-workout meal immediately afterward to aid muscle recovery.
2. **5:2 Fasting Plan**: Schedule more demanding strength training sessions on your normal eating days to take advantage of higher calorie availability. On lower-calorie days, opt for gentle yoga or a leisurely walk to stay active without overexerting yourself.

By understanding and implementing these strategies, you can optimize your workout schedule to align perfectly with your intermittent fasting routine, enhancing your overall health and achieving your fitness goals more effectively. Remember, the key is to listen to your body and be willing to adapt as needed, ensuring that your exercise routine supports your body's needs at every stage of your fasting journey.

7.5 AVOIDING OVEREXERTION: LISTENING TO YOUR BODY'S SIGNALS

As you weave exercise into your fasting regime, it's like tuning into a new radio frequency. You're learning to listen more intently to the signals your body sends, ensuring the music of movement harmonizes with the rhythms of rest and recovery. Recognizing the signs of overexertion is crucial at this stage of life, as pushing too hard can lead to setbacks rather than health gains. It's not uncommon to experience excessive fatigue, prolonged recovery times, or a noticeable dip in performance if you're overdoing it. These signals are your body's way of asking for a gentler approach or more time to recharge.

Excessive fatigue, for instance, extends beyond the normal tiredness felt after a good workout. It lingers, seeping into your day-to-day activities, making it hard to muster energy for even small tasks. Prolonged recovery time is another red flag; it's normal to feel sore a day or two after a workout, but if the soreness persists or if your muscles feel weak long after your exercises, it might be a sign that your body hasn't fully recuperated. Decreased performance is similarly telling. If you find that your usual routine suddenly feels much more challenging, or if your endurance and strength seem to have regressed, it could be your body urging you to pull back and allow more time for recovery.

Balancing the intensity of your workouts with adequate recovery time is essential, especially when you're fasting. Your body repairs itself and strengthens during the rest periods, not while you're lifting weights or running. This balance is even more pivotal during fasting, as your body also manages energy reserves differently. Consider integrating active recovery days into your exercise plan to maintain this balance. Activities like gentle yoga, leisurely walks, or even dynamic stretching can keep you moving and aid your recovery without overtaxing your system. Think of these lighter days as part of your training; they are there to enhance your body's ability to perform and not detract from it.

Adapting your exercise plans based on how you feel daily can also prevent overexertion. This adaptive approach might mean swapping a high-intensity interval training (HIIT) session for a brisk walk if you're feeling drained, or it might involve taking an extra rest day if your body cues are telling you to pause. Remember, more isn't always better. Quality trumps quantity, especially when maintaining an exercise routine that supports your fasting lifestyle and overall well-being.

Consulting with fitness or health professionals can provide an additional layer of insight, especially when you're unsure about the signals your body is sending. A fitness coach, for example, can help tailor your exercise routine to better align with your fasting schedule and energy levels, ensuring that you're working out in a way that enhances, rather than depletes, your health. Similarly, if you're consistently feeling signs of overexertion, a visit to your healthcare provider can help determine if there's a deeper issue at play. These professionals can offer guidance that is customized to your health status, age, and fitness goals, providing a supportive framework as you navigate the integration of exercise with intermittent fasting.

Incorporating these strategies not only helps prevent the pitfalls of overexertion but also enriches your fitness journey, making it sustainable and enjoyable. By listening attentively to your body's signals, adjusting your workout intensity, incorporating sufficient recovery, and seeking professional advice when necessary, you are setting a solid foundation for long-term health and vitality. This approach ensures that your physical activities bolster your fasting efforts, enhancing your overall wellness and keeping you active and agile in the coming years.

7.6 INCORPORATING REGULAR MOVEMENT INTO YOUR ROUTINE

Embracing movement throughout your day can transform the way you feel and function, especially as you navigate the intricacies of intermittent fasting. It's not just about scheduled exercise sessions; it's about weaving activity into the very fabric of your daily life to enhance circulation, elevate your mood, and increase your overall energy expenditure. This approach ensures that staying active isn't a chore but a natural part of your day that you look forward to and enjoy.

The benefits of integrating more movement into your day are multifaceted. For starters, regular movement helps improve circulation, which is vital for maintaining heart health and ensuring that your muscles receive the nutrients they need to function optimally. Enhanced circulation also aids in the faster removal of waste products from your body, which can help reduce inflammation and decrease the risk of chronic diseases. Additionally, frequent physical activity is a known mood booster. It stimulates the production of endorphins, often referred to as 'feel-good' hormones, which can naturally elevate your mood and combat feelings of stress or anxiety—a common concern during fasting periods. Moreover, incorporating movement throughout your day naturally increases your calorie burn, which can be particularly beneficial if weight management is one of your goals with intermittent fasting.

Simple Ways to Increase Daily Movement

Incorporating more activity into your daily routine doesn't have to mean lengthy sessions at the gym or exhaustive runs. Simple, deliberate choices to move more can be equally effective. For instance, opting for the stairs instead of the elevator is a quick way to increase your heart rate and strengthen your leg muscles. Similarly, if you find yourself on long phone calls, consider walking while you talk. Not only does this break the monotony of sitting, but it also adds a considerable amount of steps to your day. Another practical tip is to set regular movement reminders on your phone or computer, especially if you have a desk job. These reminders can prompt you to stand up, stretch, or do a quick series of exercises like squats or wall push-ups, helping to keep your metabolism active and your body engaged.

Incorporating Activity into Lifestyle

To make physical activity a seamless part of your lifestyle, choose forms of movement that you genuinely enjoy. If you love music, perhaps a dance class could be a delightful way to get your heart pumping. Or, if you find peace in the outdoors, gardening can be a therapeutic way to stay active, bending, and stretching as you tend to plants and flowers. Playing with grandchildren or joining a community sports team can also be wonderful ways to stay active while engaging with loved ones or making new friends. The key is associating physical activity with pleasure rather than duty, making it something you look forward to rather than a box to tick off your daily to-do list.

Setting and Tracking Movement Goals

To keep motivated and on track with your movement goals, using a pedometer or a smartphone app to monitor your steps can be incredibly effective. Setting daily or weekly goals, such as achieving a certain number of steps or dedicating a specific amount of time to physical activity, can give you a clear target to aim for. Monitoring your progress helps maintain motivation and provides a sense of accomplishment as you meet and exceed your goals. For instance, you might start with a goal of 5,000 steps per day, gradually increasing this as your fitness improves. Celebrating these small victories can significantly boost your morale and encourage you to keep moving, enhancing your overall health and well-being.

Incorporating regular movement into your routine is essential to a healthy lifestyle, especially when paired with intermittent fasting. Finding joy in everyday activities, setting achievable goals, and tracking your progress ensures that staying active is a delightful, rewarding part of your daily life. This chapter closes with a gentle reminder that movement, in any form, celebrates your body's capabilities and is a testament to your commitment to maintaining vibrant health as you navigate the later years of life with grace and vitality. As we transition to the next chapter, we will explore strategies for sustaining your intermittent fasting and fitness efforts long-term, ensuring that the changes you've embraced are not fleeting but become a permanent and cherished part of your lifestyle.

LONG-TERM STRATEGIES FOR SUCCESS

Imagine your life as a beautifully woven tapestry, each thread representing a different aspect of your daily routine, your habits, and the choices you make. Intermittent fasting, when introduced into this fabric, isn't just a thread running alongside others; it gradually intertwines with them, becoming an integral part of your life's design. This chapter is about reinforcing that integration, ensuring that intermittent fasting isn't just a practice you adopt temporarily but a sustainable part of your lifestyle that enhances your health and happiness for years to come.

8.1 DEVELOPING A LONG-TERM MINDSET: BEYOND QUICK FIXES

Embarking on the intermittent fasting path can often start with a burst of enthusiasm—eager for quick results; you might dive in headfirst. However, true and lasting benefits come from viewing intermittent fasting as a long-term health journey rather than a quick-fix solution to immediate issues like weight or health concerns. It's about nurturing a deep-seated shift in how you relate to food and your body, which takes time and patience.

Understanding the difference between sustainability and quick results is crucial. Intermittent fasting offers numerous health benefits, such as improved metabolism, better blood sugar control, enhanced brain function, and increased fat loss. However, these changes occur over time and with consistent practice. The body needs time to adjust to new eating patterns, and the mind must adopt new habits and leave behind old ones, which doesn't happen overnight. Embrace this transition's slow and steady nature, recognizing that each day contributes to a larger goal.

Setting realistic, measurable, and time-bound goals is essential for maintaining motivation and tracking progress. Start with clear, manageable goals that align with your long-term health aspirations. For example, instead of aiming to lose a certain amount of weight quickly, set goals for gradual weight loss over several months or seek to improve your blood markers, like cholesterol levels or blood pressure, by your next annual check-up. These goals should evolve as you progress, adapting to your changing health needs and circumstances.

Patience and persistence are your allies in this journey. There will be days when you feel like you are not making progress or when life's circumstances make it challenging to stick to your fasting schedule. It's normal to experience setbacks or feel frustrated. However, the key is to persist, learn from each experience, and continue moving forward. Celebrate small successes along the way —perhaps you skipped a late-night snack, made a healthier meal choice, or simply felt more energetic during the day. These small victories accumulate, reinforcing your commitment and helping you see the tangible benefits of your efforts.

Integrating intermittent fasting into your daily life so that it feels like a natural part of your routine is perhaps the most crucial step. This might mean aligning your eating windows with your social life or work schedule to make fasting feel less like a disruption. It could also involve incorporating family and friends into your journey, perhaps by sharing meals during your eating windows or discussing the benefits you're experiencing, which not only enhances your support system but also normalizes your new lifestyle choice. The aim is to weave intermittent fasting so seamlessly into your life that it no longer feels like a special effort but rather just another part of your day.

Incorporating intermittent fasting as a permanent aspect of your lifestyle ensures that it supports your physical health, overall well-being, and life satisfaction. By developing a long-term mindset, setting evolving goals, practicing patience, and integrating fasting into your daily life, you transform intermittent fasting from a mere diet trend into a sustainable lifestyle that nurtures your body and enriches your life. As you continue to adapt and refine your approach, intermittent fasting becomes not just something you do but a part of who you are—contributing to a fuller, healthier future.

8.2 ADAPTING IF PRACTICES AS YOU AGE

As the years gracefully add up, embracing the changes that come with age becomes crucial to maintaining your health and well-being. It's much like adjusting your sail to the ever-changing wind; as your body evolves, so too should your approach to intermittent fasting. Recognizing and adapting to these changes is not just about perseverance; it's about smart, responsive adjustments that honor your body's current needs.

The metabolic rate—how fast your body converts food into energy—naturally slows down as you age. This slowdown is a result of several factors, including loss of muscle mass, hormonal changes, and alterations in cellular function. While these changes might sound daunting, understanding them empowers you to make informed adjustments to your intermittent fasting routine, ensuring it remains effective and comfortable. For instance, as metabolism slows, you might find that shorter fasting periods or less frequent extended fasts are more suitable. This adjustment helps maintain energy levels and manage weight, as your body may not be as efficient at processing large meals or bouncing back from long fasting windows as it used to be.

Adjusting fasting windows and frequency is more art than science, requiring you to listen closely to your body's feedback. Start by slightly shortening your fasting periods if you find yourself feeling more fatigued than usual or if weight management becomes a struggle. Alternatively, increasing the frequency of your fasting days might be beneficial if your daily caloric needs decrease. However, you still want to enjoy a variety of foods during your eating windows. It's about finding that sweet spot where you feel energized and satisfied without overwhelming your body. Regular experimentation and adjustments can help you maintain an effective fasting schedule that adapts to your changing metabolic rate and lifestyle.

Regular health check-ups become increasingly crucial as you integrate intermittent fasting into your later years. These check-ups provide valuable insights into how your body is responding to fasting. For example, monitoring blood glucose levels, cholesterol, and blood pressure can help gauge the effectiveness of your fasting routine in managing or improving these markers. Moreover, regular check-ups can catch potential health issues early, allowing for timely adjustments to your fasting plan. This proactive approach ensures that your intermittent fasting practice supports your health without inadvertently causing issues.

Listening to your body is perhaps the most personal and direct way to adapt your fasting practices as you age. Pay attention to how you feel during different fasting windows and note any changes in your energy levels, mood, and physical comfort. Your body communicates through symptoms like increased fatigue, irritability, or digestive discomfort, signaling when it's time to tweak your fasting routine. Being attuned to these signals allows you to customize your intermittent fasting approach, aligning it closely with your body's needs. This might mean adjusting the timing of your meals to earlier in the day when you feel more energetic or allowing yourself a bit more flexibility on days when energy is low.

Adapting your intermittent fasting practices as you age is not about sticking rigidly to a routine that worked for you five or ten years ago. It's about evolving your approach to suit your current physical condition and health needs. By understanding the metabolic changes that come with age, adjusting your fasting windows and frequency, staying on top of health check-ups, and listening to your body's signals, you ensure that intermittent fasting continues to be a beneficial and sustainable part of your lifestyle. This adaptive, responsive approach not only supports your physical health but also enhances your overall quality of life, allowing you to enjoy your later years with vitality and grace.

8.3 KEEPING A JOURNAL: TRACKING YOUR PROGRESS AND REFLECTIONS

Keeping a journal as you navigate through your intermittent fasting experience isn't just about jotting down what you ate or when you fasted. It's a powerful tool that helps you tune into your body's rhythms, understand your emotional and physical responses, and recognize patterns that emerge over time. Think of your journal as a map that helps you navigate your own personal landscape of wellness. By documenting your journey, you create a feedback loop that not only tracks your progress but also deepens your understanding of how intermittent fasting affects you, both physically and emotionally.

The benefits of maintaining a detailed journal are manifold. Firstly, it allows you to track your progress in a structured way, helping you to see how far you've come since you began. This can be incredibly motivating, especially on days when progress feels slow or invisible. Moreover, your journal can help you identify how different fasting schedules affect your mood, energy levels, and overall well-being. You might discover, for instance, that shorter fasting periods leave you feeling more energetic or that your mood dips on days when you start your fast later in the day. These insights are invaluable as they guide you to tailor your fasting regime in ways that best support your health and lifestyle.

In your journal, consider recording several aspects of your intermittent fasting journey. Start with the basics, like fasting durations and the timing of your eating windows. Note what you eat during your feeding periods to ensure you're not only sticking to your fasting schedule but also making nutritious choices that support your fasting efforts. It's also essential to track your physical responses—any changes in weight, alterations in sleep patterns, or physical symptoms like headaches or nausea. Equally crucial are your emotional reactions. How do you feel during and after fasting? Are there changes in your stress levels or overall mood? Documenting these details can help you make connections between your fasting protocol and your physical and emotional health.

Using the information from your journal requires a bit of reflection. Set aside some time each week to review your entries. Look for trends or patterns that emerge. Are there particular days of the week you find it harder to stick to your fasting schedule? Do specific foods during your eating windows improve energy levels the following day? This review process can highlight what's working and what might need adjustment. For instance, if you notice that your energy levels consistently dip after a heavy meal at the end of your eating window, you might consider adjusting your meal composition or timing.

Journaling also serves as a foundation for reflective practices that enhance your mental and emotional well-being. Consider incorporating gratitude logging, where you note things you're thankful for each day. This practice can shift your focus from any challenges you're facing to the positive aspects of your life, enhancing your overall resilience and emotional health. Another reflective practice is noting learning points at the end of each day or week. What did you learn about your body's needs? What insights did you gain about your relationship with food? These reflections can deepen your understanding of yourself and your fasting journey, fostering a sense of personal growth and self-awareness.

Ultimately, your journal is a personal space for exploration and reflection. It's a tool that helps you monitor your intermittent fasting journey and connects you with your deeper health and wellness goals. By regularly documenting and reviewing your experiences, you create a dynamic record of your journey that tracks your progress and celebrates your commitment to living a healthier, more mindful life. As you continue to update your journal, you'll likely find that it becomes not just a systematic record but a story of transformation—one that you are both authoring and living, day by day.

8.4 COMMUNITY AND SUPPORT: FINDING LIKE-MINDED INDIVIDUALS

Navigating the path of intermittent fasting can sometimes feel like a solo journey, but it doesn't have to be. Just as a tree thrives in a forest, drawing strength from its surroundings, immersing yourself in a supportive community can significantly enhance your fasting experience. The importance of a robust support system cannot be overstated—it provides motivation shared knowledge and emotional support that can make all the difference during challenging times.

Finding and engaging with like-minded individuals can transform your intermittent fasting practice from a solitary endeavor into a shared experience, enriching it with diverse perspectives and encouragement. Start by exploring both local and online intermittent fasting communities. Online platforms, social media groups, and forums offer a treasure trove of resources where experiences, tips, and motivational stories are exchanged. Websites like Meetup can be instrumental in finding local groups focused on intermittent fasting or broader wellness and health topics. These groups often organize regular meetings, which can be an excellent way to connect with others who are also exploring similar lifestyle changes. Engaging in online or in-person discussions can provide new insights and reaffirm that you are part of a vibrant, supportive community.

If local options are limited or existing groups don't quite meet your needs, consider starting your own intermittent fasting group. This could be among friends, family members, or colleagues who have shown interest in your lifestyle changes. Organizing a small, informal group provides a sense of ownership and allows you to tailor activities and discussions to align closely with your group's interests and goals. It could be as simple as a monthly breakfast where the focus is discussing challenges and successes, sharing recipes, or even inviting a guest speaker to learn more about nutrition and health.

Active participation in these communities plays a crucial role. Sharing your own experiences and tips not only helps others but also reinforces your own understanding and commitment to intermittent fasting. It's a reciprocal relationship; the more you put in, the more you and the entire group benefit. Engaging actively also builds a sense of belonging and accountability, which can be incredibly motivating. For instance, if you learned a new recipe that fits well within your eating window, sharing it with your group can spark conversations about nutrition and meal planning that benefit everyone. Similarly, if you encounter a challenge and find a way to overcome it, discussing this can provide encouragement and practical strategies that others might find useful.

This sense of community and shared journey in intermittent fasting not only helps you stick to your goals but also makes the process more enjoyable and meaningful. Each story shared, each piece of advice given, and every bit of support offered adds layers of depth and connection to your own experience, transforming intermittent fasting from a mere dietary approach into a shared journey of wellness and discovery. As you continue to connect with others, remember that every interaction is an opportunity to learn and grow together, making each step of your intermittent fasting path richer and more supported.

8.5 CONTINUOUS LEARNING: KEEPING UP-TO-DATE WITH IF RESEARCH

In the ever-evolving world of health and wellness, staying informed about the latest research in intermittent fasting, especially concerning aging populations, is akin to keeping your garden well-tended; it ensures that your practices are effective, nurturing, and safe. As new studies and data emerge, they can shed light on better ways to adapt fasting to your lifestyle, potentially offering more profound health benefits or simplifying your routine. This continuous learning process keeps your approach fresh and aligned with the latest scientific insights, empowering you to make informed decisions about your health routine.

Navigating the vast sea of information available today requires a discerning eye. Not all sources are created equal, and understanding how to critically evaluate the credibility of research studies and health information is crucial. Start by looking at the source of the information. Reputable medical journals, well-established health organizations, and universities are typically reliable sources. Be wary of articles or studies that do not cite their sources or that are published on platforms with commercial interests without peer review. Learning to distinguish between scientifically backed information and anecdotal evidence or personal testimonials is essential. While individual stories can be inspiring and provide a human element to the fasting narrative, they do not replace empirical evidence from well-conducted research studies.

Applying new knowledge from your research to your intermittent fasting practice involves careful consideration. For instance, a new study might suggest that adjusting the timing of your eating window could enhance metabolic health or improve sleep quality. Before making any changes, consider how these findings align with your current health status, fasting experience, and lifestyle needs. Discussing significant changes with a healthcare professional may be beneficial, especially if you have underlying health conditions or if the study suggests a drastic departure from current fasting methods. Healthcare professionals can provide personalized advice, helping you interpret how new research applies to your specific circumstances and whether it's a safe and beneficial option for you to consider.

Furthermore, engaging with new research can also serve as a powerful motivational tool. Learning about the mechanisms behind how intermittent fasting affects cellular health, for instance, can renew your commitment to your fasting schedule and inspire you to stick with it. Understanding the science can make the process more engaging and intellectually satisfying, which is particularly important when the physical results of fasting may be slow to manifest. For those who enjoy sharing their knowledge with others, discussing new research findings in community forums or with your fasting support group can reinforce your understanding and help others who may benefit from the information.

Staying updated with the latest intermittent fasting research ensures that your practice is supported by the most current scientific understanding, enhancing its effectiveness and sustainability. By learning to critically evaluate sources, applying new knowledge judiciously, and using this information to stay motivated, you ensure that your intermittent fasting practice remains a dynamic and informed response to your evolving health needs. This approach deepens your understanding and enriches your overall experience, keeping you engaged and proactive about your health journey.

8.6 WHEN TO REEVALUATE YOUR IF APPROACH

As you continue to weave intermittent fasting into the fabric of your life, it's like nurturing a garden; it requires regular attention and occasional adjustments to thrive. Knowing when to step back and reassess your approach to fasting is crucial, as it ensures that your routine continues to align with your evolving needs and lifestyle. Think of this process as a periodic tune-up that helps keep your vehicle—the body—running smoothly on its path to wellness.

One clear sign that it's time to reevaluate your fasting approach is persistent fatigue. It's normal to feel a bit tired when first adjusting to a new fasting schedule, but continuous or severe tiredness is a signal that your body might not be getting the energy it needs or that the stress of fasting could be too much at the moment. Similarly, if you're not seeing the results you anticipated or if your health markers have plateaued or worsened, these are indicators that adjustments might be necessary. Changes in health status, such as new diagnoses or changes in your physical condition, also warrant a re-examination of your fasting plan to ensure that it remains beneficial and safe.

When these signs appear, it's wise to consult with dietary or medical professionals. These experts can provide a fresh perspective and specialized knowledge that is crucial in effectively reassessing and modifying your fasting plan. For instance, a nutritionist can help optimize your meal plans during eating windows to ensure you're getting adequate nutrients, while a physician might advise on adjusting the length of your fasts to better suit your medical conditions or medications.

Experimenting with adjustments to your fasting schedule, diet composition, and other lifestyle factors is a natural part of this re-evaluation process. Changing your eating window or trying a different fasting method could rekindle progress and alleviate issues. It's important, however, to make these adjustments gradually and monitor how they affect you. This cautious approach helps prevent negative effects and makes it easier to identify which changes are beneficial. Remember, what works best for someone else might not be ideal for you, so this experimentation should be personalized and considered.

A holistic assessment of well-being extends beyond the physical aspects. It's essential to consider how intermittent fasting impacts your mental and emotional states. Are you feeling more stressed or anxious? Do you feel in control of your fasting routine, or does it dominate your daily life? These questions are important because your mental and emotional health significantly affects your overall success with intermittent fasting. If fasting is causing considerable stress or if it feels like a burden, it might be time to adjust your approach. This might mean shortening your fasting periods, shifting your fasting days to less busy times, or even allowing yourself more flexibility in general.

As you navigate through these adjustments, remember that intermittent fasting aims to enhance your life, not complicate it. It should feel like a positive, enriching part of your routine that contributes to your overall well-being. By staying attentive to the signs that suggest a need for change, consulting with professionals for guidance, experimenting with thoughtful adjustments, and considering your holistic well-being, you ensure that intermittent fasting remains a beneficial and enjoyable part of your health routine. This proactive and mindful approach not only helps you maintain an effective fasting practice but also supports a balanced and fulfilling lifestyle.

As we wrap up this chapter on reevaluating your intermittent fasting approach, we see how crucial it is to remain flexible and responsive to your body's and lifestyle's changing needs. This continual adjustment ensures that your fasting routine supports your health goals at every stage, fostering long-term success and well-being. Moving forward, we'll explore how to maintain this adaptive approach, ensuring that intermittent fasting remains a valuable tool in your wellness toolkit.

SUCCESS STORIES AND INSPIRATIONAL INSIGHTS

If you've ever wondered if intermittent fasting is just another passing trend, the stories of women like you, thriving and transforming their lives through IF, will surely dispel those doubts. Like a garden that blooms more splendidly with the right care, these women have nurtured their bodies and spirits with intermittent fasting, cultivating health, vitality, and a renewed zest for life post-50. This chapter celebrates their journeys, sharing the rich tapestry of experiences that illustrate the profound impact of IF on real lives.

9.1 TRANSFORMATIVE TALES: WOMEN OVER 50 WHO THRIVED WITH IF

Imagine sitting down with a group of friends, each sharing a story of transformation that feels both extraordinary and incredibly relatable. These are the stories of women who embraced intermittent fasting in their golden years, finding in it a key to unlocking a healthier, fuller life. Each tale is a beacon of hope and a testament to the resilience and adaptability of women like you.

Sarah, a retired school teacher from Vermont, initially struggled with weight gain and lethargy after her retirement. Her journey with IF began somewhat reluctantly, coaxed into it by her daughter, who was worried about her declining health. The first few weeks were challenging; old habits die hard, and the adjustment was not comfortable. But Sarah was no stranger to challenges. With determination, she fine-tuned her fasting schedule, aligning it with her natural rhythms and social calendar. Not only did she shed the stubborn weight, but she also discovered an unexpected surge in her energy levels. Sarah now leads a weekly hiking group for seniors in her community, sharing her love for the outdoors. "Intermittent fasting gave me back my zest for life," she shares, hoping her story inspires others to take that first step.

Then there's Lisa, who lives in sunny Florida. Diagnosed with type 2 diabetes in her late forties, Lisa faced the all-too-common battle with managing her blood sugar levels. The turning point came when her endocrinologist suggested intermittent fasting as part of her management plan. Skeptical at first, Lisa began with an easy 12-hour overnight fast. Over months, not only did her blood sugar levels stabilize, but she also experienced a significant improvement in her mental clarity—a change she hadn't anticipated but greatly cherished. "IF helped me regain control, not just over my diabetes, but over my whole health," Lisa explains, her story a powerful reminder of the holistic benefits of well-managed fasting.

Among these narratives, there's also Jenna, a freelance writer from Oregon, who turned to intermittent fasting to manage her menopausal symptoms. The hot flashes, night sweats, and mood swings were making her miserable. Intermittent fasting wasn't a miracle cure, but it brought noticeable improvements. More importantly, it led Jenna to make healthier food choices and become more active, integrating yoga and meditation into her daily routine. "It's about the whole lifestyle," Jenna notes, "IF was the catalyst for me to live more consciously and healthily."

These stories, each unique yet underscored by a common theme of transformation, highlight not just the weight loss often associated with intermittent fasting but its role in enhancing overall quality of life. By integrating IF with increased physical activity and mindful nutrition, these women have improved their physical health and enriched their lives in ways they did not anticipate. They are inspiring examples of how adopting intermittent fasting can lead to profound personal growth and well-being.

Their words of encouragement resonate deeply, each quote a nugget of wisdom gained through personal experience. "Start where you are, use what you have, do what you can," Sarah advises. Lisa urges, "Be patient with yourself. Change doesn't happen overnight, but it does happen." Jenna's call to action, "Listen to your body; it knows what it needs," reminds us of the importance of tuning into our own physical and emotional cues.

Through these narratives, you are invited not only to witness these transformations but to see the possibilities for your own life. Each story is a thread in the broader tapestry of shared experience, woven together by the common threads of challenge, adjustment, and triumph. As you read these tales, consider your own journey, your own potential for renewal and growth. Let these stories inspire you to embrace intermittent fasting not just as a dietary choice, but as a pathway to a more vibrant, healthful, and fulfilling life.

9.2 EXPERT OPINIONS: WHY DOCTORS RECOMMEND IF FOR AGING WOMEN

When considering a lifestyle change as significant as adopting intermittent fasting, it's comforting to know that this practice comes highly recommended by a chorus of medical professionals specializing in women's health, geriatrics, and nutrition. These experts don't just follow the trends; their endorsements are grounded in robust scientific reasoning that underscores the effectiveness of intermittent fasting, especially for women over 50. As you contemplate integrating IF into your routine, understanding why medical professionals advocate for this approach can provide the reassurance and confidence you need to take that step.

Dr. Elizabeth Nguyen, a renowned geriatric specialist, explains, "Intermittent fasting isn't just about weight management. For aging women, the benefits extend to enhanced metabolic health and hormonal balance, crucial factors that impact quality of life post-menopause." She highlights how IF can help regulate insulin sensitivity, which often becomes problematic as women age. Improved insulin sensitivity can reduce the risk of type 2 diabetes, a common concern among older women. Additionally, fasting has been shown to influence hormone levels positively, helping to mitigate some of the typical symptoms associated with menopause, such as hot flashes and night sweats.

The scientific rationale behind these endorsements is compelling. Studies have shown that intermittent fasting can lead to improved lipid profiles and reduced inflammation markers, both of which contribute to better cardiovascular health. Dr. Nguyen points out that "the cardiovascular risks increase significantly after menopause, and managing these risks is crucial for long-term health." Furthermore, intermittent fasting activates cellular mechanisms like autophagy, which plays a role in cell renewal and repair. This process is particularly beneficial as it can help slow down some degenerative aging processes.

However, women in their fifties and beyond often express concerns about adopting intermittent fasting, wondering if it's suitable for their age or about potential health risks. Addressing these concerns, nutritionist Dr. Sarah Lin explains, "One common worry is nutrient intake. There's a misconception that fasting leads to nutritional deficiencies." She reassures that with careful planning and guidance, women can maintain a balanced diet that supports their fasting schedule. Dr. Lin also addresses concerns about energy levels, noting that "while there might be an initial period of adjustment, many of my patients report higher energy levels and better mental clarity once they adapt to their new eating patterns."

For those considering intermittent fasting, integrating it with medical guidance is crucial. "It's not a one-size-fits-all approach," states Dr. Nguyen. She recommends that women work closely with their healthcare providers to tailor fasting protocols that fit their specific health needs, lifestyle, and medical conditions. This personalized approach ensures that the fasting routine supports their health without compromising it. For instance, women with thyroid issues or diabetes require careful monitoring and adjustments to their fasting schedules to ensure their conditions are managed safely.

Integrative Approach

To illustrate, Dr. Nguyen shares the story of a patient, Marianne, who successfully integrated intermittent fasting into her health plan for managing hypertension. "Marianne was initially hesitant," she recalls, "but by working closely together, adjusting her medication timings, and monitoring her response to fasting, we found a rhythm that worked beautifully for her." This integrative approach not only helped Marianne manage her blood pressure more effectively but also improved her overall well-being.

This collaborative, informed, and cautious approach to intermittent fasting can make all the difference, turning it from a mere diet trend into a sustainable lifestyle change that enhances your health and vitality. As these medical professionals highlight, with the right guidance and a clear understanding of the scientific principles behind IF, aging women can safely and effectively incorporate this practice into their lives, reaping benefits that go far beyond weight loss.

9.3 OVERCOMING HEALTH HURDLES WITH INTERMITTENT FASTING

Navigating the path of intermittent fasting (IF) is not just about adjusting eating windows or managing hunger; for many, it's a profound transformation in managing chronic health conditions. The beauty of IF lies in its flexibility, allowing it to be tailored to meet different health challenges, particularly those that tend to surface as we age, such as type 2 diabetes, high blood pressure, and elevated cholesterol levels. The stories of those who have turned these health challenges around with IF are not just inspiring; they are a testament to the adaptability and efficacy of this approach.

Take, for example, the story of Anne, a 58-year-old who was grappling with escalating blood pressure and cholesterol levels. Her journey with intermittent fasting started out of a necessity to manage these issues without relying heavily on medications. Under the guidance of her healthcare provider, Anne started with a mild 14/10 fasting schedule, which means fasting for 14 hours and eating over a 10-hour window. This gentle introduction helped her body adapt without significant stress. Over time, as her body responded positively, she and her doctor decided to gradually increase her fasting intervals. This adaptive strategy was key in not just meeting but exceeding her health goals. Anne's blood pressure and cholesterol levels improved remarkably, and she found herself reducing her medications. "IF has given me a new lease on life where I feel in control of my health," Anne reflects, hoping her story can encourage others to see beyond the dietary aspect of IF and appreciate its potential in chronic disease management.

Similarly, the experience of James, who has been battling type 2 diabetes, highlights how IF can be integrated into existing health management plans to enhance outcomes. James started intermittent fasting with a lot of skepticism, worried about how it might affect his blood sugar levels. With professional support, he began a tailored IF protocol that included monitoring his blood sugar levels multiple times throughout his fasting periods. This careful, personalized approach allowed for real-time adjustments. Over months, James not only saw a significant stabilization in his blood sugar levels but also a reduction in his dependence on insulin. His doctor was particularly impressed by the improvement in his A1C levels, a key indicator of long-term blood glucose management. James believes that "IF isn't just a diet; it's a tool that's helped me reclaim my health from diabetes."

The role of healthcare providers in these stories cannot be overstressed. Their expertise in tailoring IF approaches to individual health profiles ensures not only the effectiveness of the routine but also its safety. Collaborating closely with healthcare providers helped individuals like Anne and James navigate their health challenges more effectively, making adjustments that were informed by medical knowledge and real-time health data. This professional support is crucial, particularly when using IF to manage chronic conditions, as it ensures that the routine complements other treatments and lifestyle changes.

For those facing similar health hurdles, let these stories remind you of the potential that IF holds. It's not merely about losing weight or managing your eating schedule—it's a potentially transformative practice that can significantly impact how you manage and potentially improve chronic conditions. As you consider or continue with intermittent fasting, remember the importance of flexibility in your approach and the value of professional guidance. Each person's health journey is unique, and the adaptability of IF can be a powerful ally in addressing personal health challenges. Whether you are dealing with a chronic condition or looking to prevent health issues in the future, intermittent fasting offers a promising avenue, backed by both personal success stories and growing scientific research, to explore in your quest for better health.

9.4 MENTAL HEALTH IMPROVEMENTS FROM REAL IF PRACTITIONERS

Imagine waking up feeling clear-headed, calm, and ready to embrace the day with a sense of purpose and vitality. For many women over 50, this isn't just a daydream but a reality they attribute to intermittent fasting (IF). Beyond the physical health benefits, IF holds profound implications for mental well-being, offering a gateway to enhanced cognitive function and emotional balance. The stories of women who have experienced these changes are not just uplifting; they illuminate the path for others, considering IF as a tool for mental rejuvenation.

Carol, a 62-year-old former librarian, shares her experience with intermittent fasting as a journey not just of weight loss but of significant mental clarity. Before IF, Carol struggled with foggy thinking and occasional forgetfulness, common complaints that can be distressing. After six months of a tailored IF routine, she noticed a marked improvement in her memory and concentration. "It's like the fog has lifted," Carol explains. "I can focus on my writing and engage in conversations without that frustrating search for words that used to plague me." This enhancement in cognitive function is supported by emerging research suggesting that IF can increase levels of brain-derived neurotrophic factor (BDNF). This protein plays a key role in neuron growth and protection. Increased BDNF levels are linked to improved brain health, potentially staving off cognitive decline associated with aging.

Mood regulation is another area where intermittent fasting shines, as shared by Julia, a 55-year-old yoga instructor. The hormonal fluctuations that come with menopause had left her feeling like she was on an emotional rollercoaster. "Starting IF was initially about body weight," she says, "but the impact on my mood was unexpected and profound." Julia found that the discipline of fasting helped stabilize her blood sugar levels, which, in turn, seemed to smooth out the highs and lows of her emotional states. The science backs up her experience, showing that reduced inflammation from IF can lead to better mood regulation. Chronic inflammation is often linked to mood disorders, and by decreasing inflammation, IF may help alleviate some of the mood variability that can disrupt daily life.

The personal stories of these women highlight not only the psychological benefits of IF but also practical strategies for maximizing these advantages. For instance, timing your fasting to align with natural circadian rhythms can enhance the cognitive benefits of IF. Carol prefers to start her fast after dinner and break it in the late morning, aligning her eating window with times when she needs the most mental energy. She also emphasizes the importance of hydration during fasting periods, which helps maintain cognitive function and prevent the brain fog that can come with dehydration.

Integrating mindfulness practices with IF is another highly recommended strategy by those who have found mental clarity through fasting. Julia incorporates meditation and gentle yoga into her fasting routine, practices that complement the mental health benefits of IF by reducing stress and enhancing overall mindfulness. "The combination of IF and mindfulness keeps me centered," she shares, "It's a holistic approach that treats mind and body as interconnected."

These personal testimonies not only underscore the cognitive and emotional benefits of IF but also offer a beacon of hope and practical advice for others looking to enhance their mental well-being. As you explore the potential of intermittent fasting to improve not just your body but also your mind, remember that the journey is highly personal. What works for one may not work for another, and the key is to tailor the fasting approach to fit your unique lifestyle and mental health needs. By doing so, you open up a world of possibilities where enhanced mental clarity and emotional balance are within reach, empowering you to lead a more fulfilling and engaged life as you navigate the complexities of your fifties and beyond.

9.5 THE ROLE OF IF IN LONGEVITY AND DISEASE PREVENTION

When you think about aging gracefully, the conversation often steers towards maintaining an active lifestyle and eating right. But what if there was more you could do that goes beyond the typical advice? Intermittent fasting (IF) has been shining brightly on the radar of those interested in extending their lifespan and reducing the risk of age-related diseases. Groundbreaking research suggests that IF isn't just about managing weight—it's a key player in promoting longevity and preventing diseases that commonly appear later in life, such as Alzheimer's, heart disease, and osteoporosis.

The connection between IF and increased lifespan is supported by various studies that show its impact on the fundamental processes of aging. Research indicates that IF can enhance the body's ability to repair its DNA and optimize cellular function—processes that are crucial for slowing down the aging clock and enhancing longevity. One fascinating study published in the *Cell Metabolism* journal found that periodic fasting was associated with longer lifespans and a lower incidence of diseases commonly associated with aging. The researchers observed that IF influenced several biological pathways that are known to regulate lifespan. These include improved metabolic efficiency and body composition, reduced oxidative stress, and lower inflammation levels—factors that are directly linked to aging and chronic diseases.

Focusing on the preventative aspects of IF, it's compelling to see how this eating pattern helps ward off illnesses that are prevalent as we age. The mechanisms through which IF exerts its effects are complex and multifaceted. One of the key mechanisms is autophagy, a process that involves the body's cellular cleanup services. During fasting periods, autophagy rates increase, allowing your body to break down and remove dysfunctional proteins that build up inside cells, which might otherwise contribute to Alzheimer's disease or other age-related conditions. Moreover, IF helps regulate hormones such as insulin, growth hormone, and leptin, all of which play significant roles in metabolism, body weight, and overall health. By improving hormonal balance, IF can help maintain bone density, reduce the risk of osteoporosis, and protect against cardiovascular diseases by improving heart function and lowering blood pressure.

The insights from Dr. Linda Peterson, a clinician specializing in geriatric medicine, further illuminate the preventative benefits of IF. In her practice, she has observed notable improvements in her patients who adopt intermittent fasting, particularly in managing chronic conditions and their overall vitality. "The anti-inflammatory and cardioprotective effects of intermittent fasting can significantly impact the health trajectories of older adults," Dr. Peterson notes. She often discusses with her patients how IF can be a tool not just for weight management but as a preventive strategy to support their health as they age.

Dr. Peterson also addresses a common concern among older adults—the fear that fasting might exacerbate existing health issues or lead to nutritional deficiencies. She reassures her patients by citing studies that show how controlled intermittent fasting, under medical supervision, does not generally lead to nutritional deficits but instead can lead to improved nutrient metabolism and more efficient energy use. Her approach always includes personalized adjustments to ensure that each patient's unique health needs are met, emphasizing that intermittent fasting, like any other health strategy, should be tailored to the individual.

As you consider the role of intermittent fasting in your own life, especially with an eye toward prevention and longevity, it's crucial to approach it with a mindset that embraces gradual, sustainable integration into your lifestyle. The potential benefits of IF extend far beyond mere weight control, offering a promising avenue for enhancing your health span and potentially reducing the burden of age-related diseases. Whether you're looking to revitalize your energy levels, protect your cognitive faculties, or simply age with fewer health complications, intermittent fasting presents a fascinating and research-backed option to consider.

9.6 CELEBRATING YOUR SUCCESS: EMBRACING A HEALTHIER, HAPPIER YOU

As you navigate the rewarding path of intermittent fasting, celebrating your milestones isn't just a joyful act—it's a vital part of maintaining your motivation and recognizing the hard work you've put into transforming your life. Think of these celebrations as markers along a hiking trail, each one offering a moment to stop, breathe, and appreciate how far you've come. These moments of celebration can greatly enhance your sense of accomplishment and encourage you to continue on your path with renewed energy.

One delightful way to celebrate your successes is by hosting a healthy meal with friends or family. Imagine this as your opportunity to share not just food but also the stories of your journey. Cooking a meal that aligns with your intermittent fasting lifestyle and inviting loved ones to share it with you serves multiple purposes. It allows you to showcase the delicious, nutritious recipes you've incorporated into your routine, and it also opens up a space for conversation about healthy living. This can be particularly uplifting and affirming, allowing you to reflect on your progress and share your challenges and victories with those who matter most.

Alternatively, treating yourself to a wellness retreat can be a profoundly restorative way to celebrate a significant fasting milestone. A retreat can provide a serene environment where you can reflect on your experiences, immerse yourself in tranquility, and perhaps even learn new practices that complement your fasting lifestyle, such as yoga or meditation. This time away from your daily routine not only rewards you but also reinforces your commitment to maintaining your health and well-being, providing a fresh burst of inspiration.

Reflective exercises are another cornerstone of celebrating your intermittent fasting achievements. Take some time to compare your health metrics or overall well-being at the start of your fasting journey to where you are now. This could involve looking at changes in your weight, energy levels, or even blood markers like cholesterol and blood sugar. Writing these reflections down can provide tangible proof of how far you've come, which can be incredibly motivating. It's also a way to pinpoint areas where you might want to focus next, helping you refine your approach as you continue with intermittent fasting.

Sharing your success plays a crucial role, not just in your own life but also in inspiring others. Whether it's through social media, a blog, or casual conversations, talking about your intermittent fasting journey can empower others to consider or persist with their own health goals. Your story could encourage someone else to start or keep going. Building this kind of support network helps others and strengthens your commitment, creating a community of motivation and encouragement.

As you look ahead, setting future health and wellness goals is essential to keep the momentum going. Now that you've seen what you can achieve with intermittent fasting, consider what other areas of your health and lifestyle you might explore or improve. Perhaps you want to focus more on physical activity or learn more about nutritional cooking. Setting new goals keeps the journey exciting and ensures continuous engagement with your health. Remember, each small goal you set and achieve is a building block for your long-term wellness.

Celebrating your intermittent fasting successes through gatherings, retreats, reflective exercises, sharing your journey, and setting new goals does more than just acknowledge your hard work. It knits a fabric of continuous motivation, support, and personal growth, enriching your life and potentially the lives of others. These celebrations and reflections are not just about looking back—they're about looking forward, continuously moving towards a healthier, happier you.

As this chapter closes, remember that each step in your intermittent fasting journey is a step towards not just a healthier body but a fuller, richer life. The practices and strategies discussed here are more than just components of a diet—they're parts of a holistic approach to living well. Carry these insights forward as you continue to explore and embrace the transformative power of intermittent fasting and the vibrant life it can help you lead.

CONCLUSION

As we draw the curtains on this journey together, I want to take a moment to reflect on the path we've traveled. Intermittent fasting, especially for us women over 50, isn't just a series of skipped meals —it's a gateway to a renewed sense of self and a healthier body. We've navigated through the what, why, and how of intermittent fasting, uncovering its potential to transform our lives beyond just weight loss.

From our initial exploration in Chapter 1 about the essence of intermittent fasting to diving into the various fasting methods in Chapter 3, and integrating these practices into our daily routines in Chapter 8, each step has added layers of understanding and empowerment. We've debunked myths, tackled the initial physical and mental challenges, and celebrated the profound benefits that extend beyond the scale—enhanced mental clarity, revitalized energy, and a deeper connection with our body's natural rhythms.

The transformative potential of intermittent fasting is clear—it's not merely about changing when we eat but about reshaping our relationship with food to honor our body's needs and our life's rhythms. It's about finding balance and harmony within and recognizing that each meal, each fasting period, is a step towards better health.

The holistic benefits we've discussed are just as vital. Intermittent fasting has the potential to improve our metabolism, reduce inflammation, and support our mental health, providing a foundation for a vibrant, active lifestyle. This isn't just about adding years to our lives—it's about adding life to our years, enabling us to enjoy this wonderful stage with vitality and joy.

I encourage you to keep learning and adapting as you continue on this path. The world of health and wellness is ever-evolving, and staying informed will help you refine your fasting practice to better suit your changing needs. Engage with communities, share your experiences, and perhaps even inspire others to embark on their own journey of health discovery.

Now, my call to action for you is simple yet profound:

1. Start where you are, use what you have, and do what you can.
2. Whether it's choosing a fasting window that fits your lifestyle or experimenting with different types of fasting schedules, take that first step.
3. Remember, this isn't a race; it's a journey that deserves patience and perseverance.

In closing, I want to express my heartfelt gratitude for allowing me to be a part of your journey. Whether you're just starting out or looking to deepen your practice, remember that each day presents a new opportunity to nourish your body and your soul. Let's continue to embrace these moments, to learn from them, and to grow together.

Here's to stepping forward with courage, curiosity, and a hearty appetite for life. Cheers to thriving at every age, and may your intermittent fasting journey be as fulfilling and enlightening as every sunrise that greets us.

GLOSSARY

Autophagy: The body's process of cleaning out damaged cells to regenerate newer, healthier cells.

Basal Metabolic Rate (BMR): The number of calories your body needs to perform basic life-sustaining functions at rest.

Brain-derived neurotrophic Factor (BDNF): A protein that supports the survival, development, and function of neurons.

Cardiovascular Diseases: A class of diseases that involve the heart or blood vessels, such as coronary artery disease.

Cortisol: A stress hormone that helps control blood sugar levels, regulate metabolism, and reduce inflammation.

Diabetes: A metabolic disease characterized by high blood sugar levels over a prolonged period.

Elliptical: A stationary exercise machine used to simulate stair climbing, walking, or running without causing excessive pressure on the joints.

Endocrinologist: A doctor who specializes in the glands and hormones of the body and their related disorders.

Estrogen: A primary female sex hormone responsible for regulating reproductive and other bodily functions.

Hormone Balance: The state of having hormones at optimal levels for healthy bodily function.

Hypertension: High blood pressure, a condition in which the force of the blood against the artery walls is too high.

Insulin: A hormone that regulates blood sugar levels by facilitating the uptake of glucose into cells.

Intermittent Fasting (IF): An eating pattern that cycles between periods of fasting and eating.

Legumes: A class of vegetables that includes beans, peas, and lentils, known for their high protein and fiber content.

Leptin: A hormone produced by fat cells that helps to regulate body weight by signaling the brain to reduce appetite.

Lipid Profiles, Including Cholesterol and Triglycerides: Blood tests that measure the levels of fats in your blood, including cholesterol and triglycerides.

Lipolysis: The process of breaking down fats into fatty acids and glycerol for energy.

Magnesium: A mineral crucial for many bodily functions, including muscle and nerve function, blood sugar control, and bone health.

Mental Clarity: The state of having a clear, focused, and sharp mind.

Metabolic Rates: The rate at which your body burns calories to maintain basic physiological functions.

Natural Circadian Rhythms: The 24-hour internal clock that regulates sleep-wake cycles and other physiological processes.

Norepinephrine: A hormone and neurotransmitter involved in the body's fight-or-flight response.

Osteoporosis: A condition characterized by weak and brittle bones, increasing the risk of fractures.

Phytoestrogens: Plant-derived compounds that can mimic the effects of estrogen in the body.

Plateaus: Periods during weight loss or fitness journeys where progress seems to stall or slow down.

Potassium: A vital mineral that helps maintain proper cell function, fluid balance, and nerve and muscle function.

Pranayama: A practice in yoga involving breath control techniques to improve physical and mental well-being.

Progesterone: A hormone involved in the menstrual cycle, pregnancy, and embryogenesis.

Post-Menopause: The stage in a woman's life after she has not had a menstrual period for 12 consecutive months.

Sodium: An essential mineral important for maintaining fluid balance, nerve function, and muscle contraction.

Satiety-Inducing Hormones: Hormones that signal fullness and reduce the desire to eat, such as leptin and ghrelin.

KEEPING THE GAME ALIVE

Now you have everything you need to achieve your health goals, it's time to pass on your newfound knowledge and show other readers where they can find the same help.

Simply by leaving your honest opinion of this book on Amazon, you'll show other women over 50 where they can find the information they're looking for, and pass their passion for intermittent fasting forward.

Thank you for your help. Intermittent fasting is kept alive when we pass on our knowledge – and you're helping me to do just that.

For the US

SCAN ME

For the UK

SCAN ME

REFERENCES

10 best intermittent fasting apps for weight loss. (n.d.). Good Housekeeping. Retrieved from https://www.goodhousekeeping.com/health-products/g34618367/best-apps-intermittent-fasting/

Autophagy and aging - PMC. (n.d.). Retrieved from https://www.ncbi.nlm.nih.gov/pmc/articles/PMC4644734/

A good guide to good carbs: The glycemic index. (n.d.). Harvard Health. Retrieved from https://www.health.harvard.edu/healthbeat/a-good-guide-to-good-carbs-the-glycemic-index

Avocado toast, three ways: Your new favorite recipe. (n.d.). Life by Daily Burn. Retrieved from https://dailyburn.com/life/recipes/avocado-toast-recipe/

ChatGPT (June 8, 2024) [Large language model]. (2024). OpenAI. Retrieved from [OpenAI Platform URL]

ChatGPT-generated image [Artificial intelligence image]. (2024). OpenAI. Retrieved from [OpenAI Platform URL]

Effects of intermittent energy restriction combined with a Mediterranean diet. (n.d.). Retrieved from https://www.ncbi.nlm.nih.gov/pmc/articles/PMC6627434/

Effects of intermittent fasting on health, aging, and disease. (n.d.). New England Journal of Medicine. Retrieved from https://www.nejm.org/doi/full/10.1056/NEJMra1905136

Effect of a six-week intermittent fasting intervention. (n.d.). Retrieved from https://www.ncbi.nlm.nih.gov/pmc/articles/PMC7312819/

Emotional eating and how to stop it. (n.d.). HelpGuide. Retrieved from https://www.helpguide.org/articles/diets/emotional-eating.htm

Fasting may improve health and shield against age-related diseases, study finds. (n.d.). Nutrition Insight. Retrieved from https://www.nutritioninsight.com/news/fasting-may-improve-health-and-shield-against-age-related-diseases-study-finds.html

How benzoyl peroxide cleanser & diet can help acne. (n.d.). MHT Space. Retrieved from https://mhtspace.com/lifestyle/how-benzoyl-peroxide-cleanser-diet-can-help-acne/

How intermittent fasting affects women's hormones. (n.d.). Rupa Health. Retrieved from https://www.rupahealth.com/post/how-intermittent-fasting-affects-womens-hormones

178 | REFERENCES

How to exercise safely during intermittent fasting. (n.d.). Healthline. Retrieved from https://www.healthline.com/health/how-to-exercise-safely-intermittent-fasting

Intermittent fasting and cognitive function - NCBI. (n.d.). Retrieved from https://www.ncbi.nlm.nih.gov/pmc/articles/PMC8470960/

Intermittent fasting during menopause: What do you need to know? (n.d.). Menopause Centre. Retrieved from https://www.menopausecentre.com.au/information-centre/articles/intermittent-fasting-during-menopause-what-do-you-need-to-know/

Intermittent fasting groups | Meetup. (n.d.). Retrieved from https://www.meetup.com/topics/intermittent-fasting/us/

Intermittent fasting 101 — The ultimate beginner's guide. (n.d.). Healthline. Retrieved from https://www.healthline.com/nutrition/intermittent-fasting-guide

Is intermittent fasting better than portion control? (n.d.). Skinny News. Retrieved from https://skinnynews.com/2023/09/is-intermittent-fasting-better-than-portion-control/

Learn how Kate Harrison lost weight for good with 5:2 fasting. (n.d.). Retrieved from https://kate-harrison.com/my5-2dietsuccess

Managing menopause symptoms with nutrition and diet. (n.d.). Nutrition.org.uk. Retrieved from https://www.nutrition.org.uk/nutrition-for-women/menopause/managing-menopause-symptoms-with-nutrition-and-diet/

Master intermittent fasting: 12 expert tips for wellness. (n.d.). LoseSimply. Retrieved from https://losesimply.in/expert-tips-for-mastering-intermittent-fasting/

Menopause diet: What to eat. (n.d.). BBC Good Food. Retrieved from https://www.bbcgoodfood.com/howto/guide/what-eat-menopause

Performance health & fitness centre: Women's pelvic health - Perimenopausal. (n.d.). Performance Physiotherapy. Retrieved from https://www.performancephysiotherapy.ca/Womens-Pelvic-Health/Perimenopausal

Stuffed bell peppers (Bharva Hari Mirch). (n.d.). Complete Recipes. Retrieved from https://completerecipes.com/stuffed-bell-peppers-bharva-hari-mirch.html

The definitive guide to healthy eating in your 50s and 60s. (n.d.). Healthline. Retrieved from https://www.healthline.com/nutrition/healthy-eating-wees-60s

The benefits of eating slowly and mindfully for fitness and health. (n.d.). Taylor Hutchinson Fitness. Retrieved from https://taylorhutchinsonfitness.net/the-benefits-of-eating-slowly-and-mindfully/

The effect of yoga on menopause symptoms: A randomized trial. (n.d.). PubMed. Retrieved from https://pubmed.ncbi.nlm.nih.gov/38709129/

What to know about intermittent fasting for women after 50. (n.d.). WebMD. Retrieved from https://www.webmd.com/healthy-aging/what-to-know-about-intermittent-fasting-for-women-after-50

Why keep a food diary? (n.d.). Harvard Health. Retrieved from https://www.health.harvard.edu/blog/why-keep-a-food-diary-2019013115855

7 low impact exercises for older adults to stay active. (n.d.). HumanGood. Retrieved from https://www.humangood.org/resources/senior-living-blog/low-impact-exercises-for-older-adults